Choosing a Nursing Home

Choosing a Nursing Home

Jean Baron Nassau

Funk & Wagnalls
New York

362.6
Nas

Manufactured in the United States of America
ISBN 0-308-10161-8

Library of Congress Cataloging in Publication Data

Nassau, Jean Baron.
    Choosing a nursing home.

    1. Nursing homes. I. Title [DNLM: 1. Nursing Homes—U.S.
—Popular works. WT27 AA1 N266c]
RA997.N36 1975   362.6'11'6   74-14948
ISBN 0-308-10161-8

1 2 3 4 5 6 7 8 9 10

To my children and my grandchildren,
with love and admiration

I would like to thank my good friend Victoria Tefft, Nursing Services Consultant with the New York State Department of Health, and Theodore E. DeSantis, Regional Medical Care Administration Specialist with the U.S. Department of Health, Education and Welfare for their helpful suggestions and their interest in this book; and gratefully acknowledge the staunch support and encouragement of my dear friend Dr. Don M. Wolfe.

Jean Baron Nassau

Contents

Preface

Nursing home has become a term that conjures up a sanctuary or a hell, a long-term health center for professional personalized care or a wasteland for debility and deterioration, a devotion to the needs of human beings or a dedication to profit and expansion at the sacrifice of patients.

It is only in the last few years that nursing homes have emerged from the blackness of obscurity, as hospitals did almost a century ago. A handful of people are bringing to light the maltreatment, the neglect, the atmosphere of the ancient almshouse. A handful more are making strides toward goals of legislative action and enforcement, high caliber professional health care, and genuine concern for the inherent rights of patients as individual human beings.

I have worked in the health field for over twenty years, more than a dozen of them in nursing homes. I've seen the bad, but I've seen the good, too. I've seen patients sitting in wheelchairs staring at empty walls, but I've watched and listened as other patients avidly participated in committees to run their own library or plan an outing, rehearsed their roles for a forthcoming patients' play or concert, or found satisfaction in reading to the blind or the paralyzed. I've heard the unanswered cries of patients in pain, but I've also listened to words of compassion and encouragement as a young nurse comforted and gently tended an amputee.

I am both hopeful and optimistic that one day the professional concerned nursing home will be the rule, no longer the exception. But this will never be accomplished out of wishful thinking. It will take years of deliberation and action and—perhaps most of all—the will and the determination to transform the dream into reality.

The purpose of this book is to help you to locate a nursing home of excellence, infinitely more difficult to find than a home of mediocrity; and then to understand the gamut and quality of professional care to which your patient is inherently and legally entitled. The more aware you are of your patient's lawful rights, the better equipped you will be to see that they are being recognized and met. If your efforts are matched by the efforts of others who are genuinely concerned with the welfare of their patients, then great strides can be effected toward raising the caliber of nursing homes everywhere.

During the years that I served as a nursing-home administrator, innumerable friends and acquaintances sought my advice on how to find "good" nursing homes for people they loved. I began to wonder whether or not there were any established written guidelines for the many people who found themselves in the same quandary. And so I wrote a letter to the state departments of health in all fifty states and the District of Columbia. Perhaps I took unfair advantage of those persons whose time I called upon to answer contrived questions, but I believe that the ends warranted the means.

Here is the text of the letter I wrote:

Gentlemen:

My father, who is 72 and a resident of your city, is presently in hospital, having suffered a major stroke. His doctor tells me that he will have to be placed in a nursing home, probably within the coming month.

I plan to come to _____ shortly to look for a suitable nursing home for him. Do you have any suggestions for me that will help me to find a good nursing home? Also, I would appreciate any information you can send me relative to Medicare and Medicaid benefits.

Thank you in advance for your cooperation.

Very truly yours,

The responses I received clearly illustrate the dilemma in which John Doe would find himself were he to need and solicit informed assistance.

Two states made no acknowledgment whatever.

Two states wrote that they were referring my inquiry to other agencies and that I would hear from them within a short period of time. I never heard.

Nine states sent me directories of licensed nursing homes in the state and nothing more.

Fourteen states each sent a directory and added the advice that I should contact the local social security office for information on Medicare and the local department of welfare for information on Medicaid. Of these fourteen, one advised, "Ask your father's doctor what level of care he needs, then contact those homes re openings and admissions policies." Do openings and admissions policies make a good nursing home? Another wrote that "Because we are concerned with only the licensing of facilities, we do not have information on Medicare and Medicaid benefits." No suggestions were made as to how to secure this information. A third state expressed the hope that "this letter and the directory will furnish you with the information you need."

One state advised contacting social security for Medicare and welfare for Medicaid but added nothing more, not even the directory of licensed homes that so many others found pertinent. Another referred to contacting welfare for Medicaid information but made no reference to Medicare or to any other item of information asked for in my letter.

Five of the above respondents emphasized that it was their policy not to recommend any one specific home. My letter didn't ask for that; it asked only for suggestions that would help me to make my own determination.

Three states included directories of licensed nursing homes, the referrals to social security and welfare offices, and further referral for assistance: one suggested my father's physician; another, the hospital's social service worker; and the third suggested both.

Three more states sent directories of licensed homes with referrals that omitted social security and welfare offices. One pointed to my father's doctor; another said that the hospital would take care of everything. A third suggested contacting the state nursing home association when I arrived, and sent an excellent guide on health facilities regulations published in June 1970 by the state board of health.

Three states sent no directories, but referred me to my father's physician and the hospital social service worker for information on both Medicare and Medicaid. One of the three suggested that I write to the state's nursing home association for a directory of licensed nursing homes.

Six states sent pamphlets, all of them brief but excellent. A number of them pertained to state Medicaid regulations, but there were three in particular that apply nationwide and that give valuable information in capsule form. These are *Your Medicare Handbook; Medicaid, Medicare: Which Is Which?* and *Nursing Home Care.* The first is available free at your local social security office or from the Department of Health, Education and Welfare, Social Security Administration, Baltimore, Md. 21235. The second is published by the Medical Services Administration/Social and Rehabilitation Service of the Department of Health, Education and Welfare and can be obtained from the same source or on request from some state departments of health. The third can be obtained for 25 cents from the Superintendent of Documents, U.S. Government Printing Office, Washington, D.C. 20402.

Only five states referred to my question of "Do you have any suggestions for me that will help me to find a good nursing home?" One acknowledged that "Nursing homes do vary a great deal both in services provided and in structure. I strongly recommend that a visit be made to the facility before placement." Another said the same thing in different words: "I would suggest that you personally visit any nursing home selected for consideration in order that you may make a personal evaluation of the environment, etc." Unless a nursing home is flagrantly, outrageously, and obviously neglectful of its patients, or filthy dirty, how can a layman make an evaluation if he is given no standards and no guidelines for judgment? And how is he to evaluate services or attitudes during the course of one uninformed visit?

A third state wrote that "I would suggest that when you come to _____ that you visit some nursing homes to determine where you would like your father placed (some homes are of more modern construction than others). This would imply that the date of construction is the primary factor in selecting a long-term facility for professional health care.

A letter from one state went into great detail to explain that a convalescing stroke patient would probably require physical therapy, and then named three specific homes in the general area where physical therapy was an integral part of the facilities' services. But the letter also referred to Medicare as paying the cost of nursing-home care "for a period of eligibility that could last up to 100 days or more." The letter is signed by the coordinator of the long-term care program of the division of medical facilities of the state. Apparently he is unaware that Medicare will not and cannot and does not pick up the tab for more than one hundred days of a single confinement in any nursing home (pages 96–99).

Only one state went into any detail with suggestions for locating a good home:

As to your question on how to find a good nursing home, we are not permitted, for obvious reasons, to make specific recommendations as to the relative merits of one home compared to another. However, a personal visit to some of these homes might provide you with enough information to make a decision. You would want to check on cleanliness of the home, adequacy of the nursing staff, particularly registered and licensed nurses, and quality of food served. A visit with some of the residents would be worthwhile to determine what their feelings and attitudes are toward the home and its staff. The administrator of the home should be most helpful in these matters. Your father's physician may also have some suggestions.

Finally, let me quote in toto the response received from Washington, D.C.

The attached request is returned for reason(s) checked below:

———— The fee for a copy of a birth certificate is $1.00 payable in advance. Please make your check or money order payable to the D.C. Treasurer.

———— Insufficient information for a thorough search. Please complete the form below and return it along with your check or money order.

———— Birth did not occur in Washington, D.C. Only those births occurring in the District of Columbia are registered with this office. For births occurring in other states see reverse side of this letter for correct address and fee for a certified copy. There is no single U.S. or Federal Agency which records all births on a nation-wide basis.

Very truly yours,

Chief
Vital Records Division

None of the reason(s) was "checked below." Along with the

notice was included my original letter and an application for a certified copy of a birth certificate!

I said my prayer of thanks that I wasn't dependent on advice from Washington or any of the state departments of health for placing a loved one in a nursing home that would ensure him good care and merit his faith and my own.

Then I sat down to write this book.

Choosing a Nursing Home

I

Crisis

"IT'S TIME for a nursing home."

The doctor has just pronounced his verdict for the patient you love. It may be an aged mother, a beloved spouse, a twenty-year-old son, or a lifelong friend. You're confronted with a confusion of thoughts, a host of questions, and the most intensive shopping expedition you have ever launched.

Throughout your lifetime you've shopped on countless occasions, all the way from buying lemon meringue pie or mint-flavored toothpaste to selecting a two-story house or a studio apartment. When you shop for a major item such as a car, a home, perhaps a fur coat, the chances are you do considerable comparative shopping before you write out a check. You think through your alternatives, talk them over, and come to a decision only after you are satisfied that you're making the best buy for yourself and for the one or more persons directly concerned.

Now it's time to make the best buy for your patient.

Fortunately, the sanctity of the individual is more widely recognized today then ever before. In the field of health it is a focal point of planning and teaching and an issue of increasing legislative concern. In the area of long-term health care, significant advances have been made through recreation and volunteer programs, social services, patients' councils, and other patient-oriented activities. Unfortunately, concerted action toward the full achievement of this goal is inclined to lack competence, spontaneity, and wholehearted effort.

Federal funding for health care took on new and meaningful dimensions only a decade ago, but recently these funds have been sharply reduced. The variance in operation of individual health facilities runs the full gamut from excellence to out-and-out negligence. Yet illness is common to all of us; it is inescapable. When illness demands institutionalization, it presents a crisis, a crisis not only to the patient, but also to the family members or friends who care.

In a general hospital the illness crisis takes precedence over any others. Usually the physician admits his patient to the hospital where he serves as a staff member, and the patient is confined for a comparatively short period of time. The national average stay in a general hospital is only 7.7 days (12.2 days for those over 65 years of age),[1] although, of course, it may vary from overnight to several months. But even a matter of a few months is a short time when compared to long-term confinement in a nursing home.

A study conducted in June–August 1969 by the Division of Health Resource Statistics in cooperation with the U.S. Bureau for the Census[2] showed the average length of stay in nursing homes across the country to be 2.8 years, or slightly over 33½ months, a vast difference from the 7.7 or 12.2 days of hospital

[1] *Hospital Discharge Summary,* 1972. Department of Health, Education and Welfare, Washington, D.C.

[2] *Characteristics of Residents in Nursing and Personal Care Homes, United States—June–August 1969.* Department of Health, Education and Welfare, Public Health Service. Health Services and Mental Health Administration, National Center for Health Statistics, Rockville, Md., 1973.

stay as determined just three years later. The 1969 survey covered facilities whose primary service was nursing care, and included a study of intermediate care facilities along with the study of skilled nursing facilities (Chapter 2); homes restricted to domiciliary care were not included in the study. In the same year the average stay reimbursed by Medicare was 34½ *days*, but I will pursue this further on.

At the moment I am interested in pointing up the greater emotional and social crisis faced by a patient placed in a nursing home where he can anticipate months or years or the remainder of a lifetime spent in confinement. Further, his physician may or may not be able to refer him to a good nursing home. If the doctor does know of one, he may not be associated with it and so may not be able to continue with the patient's care. Or perhaps the nursing home is located in an area that makes regular visiting so difficult for you as to be nearly impossible. Or perhaps you've heard about that nursing home and didn't like what you heard; or you've already visited someone there and didn't like what you saw.

If the patient is well enough, physically and mentally, to make his own choice or to assist you in arriving at a decision, you and he are both fortunate. The likelihood, though, is that the selection of the nursing home will be primarily up to you. Crisis has been defined as a turning point, a critical time, and an occasion that demands decision-making. Now it's probably your crisis, your opportunity to find a solution. There are many months, or years, for your patient to live with the happy or unhappy consequences of the choice that is made. Whether or not he copes successfully will have a strong bearing on your conscience and your peace of mind.

If it is of any comfort to you, you are far from alone in this dilemma. Statistics show that demands to meet health needs have doubled the number of nursing homes in our country from 6,539 in 1954 to 13,047 in 1969. In the same fifteen-year period the number of nursing home *beds* has more than quadrupled: from 172,000 in 1954 to 762,465 in 1969. The total patient population of all long-term facilities was 1,099,412 in 1970.[3]

These figures can be explained in large part by the fact that in the United States alone the number of people over 65 years of age has increased from 3 million in 1900 to 20 million in 1969, and it is expected that the number will jump to 25 million by 1985.[4] In a 1969 survey of nursing homes assisted by the Federal Housing Authority, it was reported that 90 percent of the patients were over the age of 65. These golden years (how rare it is that they are golden!) are unhappily fraught with deteriorating illness, physical handicap, senility, the inability to care for daily routine needs, or one or more of a wide assortment of valid and invalid reasons for long-term institutional care.

So there are many reasons for the giddy escalation in numbers of nursing-home patients. The old maxim of threescore years and ten is as obsolete as the nickel bus fare. During the 1960s Dr. Louis Orr, former president of the American Medical Association, stated that longevity had increased by 45 percent since the turn of the century. Although monumental strides in medicine continue to make dramatic advances in life expectancy, these later years are too commonly burdened by partial or total dependency and disability. In addition, America becomes more and more a society of youth-worshippers and producer-worshippers. We frown on the aged—and the disabled —as bothersome, interfering, useless, costly, and ultimately parasitic. Once a person's productive years have ended, it is usual that the concern of society in general and of the family in particular has dissipated along with the years.

The only explanation that can be made in defense of this attitude is the economic aspect of modern living, and this constitutes an additional reason for the constantly growing popu-

[3] *Nursing Home Fact Book 1970–1971*. American Nursing Home Association, 1972.

[4] 1970 Census Report. Bureau of the Census.

lation of nursing homes. The average family resides in a small apartment or a small house where three generations under one roof can create confusion, contention, and disruptive family living. This can be a pervasive truth; it can often be a pervasive excuse. In past generations, and in Eastern cultures, three and often four generations lived together contentedly and productively, and each generation profited from the experiences and outlook of the other. Your own motivation needs careful scrutiny.

Although the overwhelming majority of nursing-home patients are aged, the approximate 10 percent under the age of 65 still constitute a significant group with urgent and crucial needs of their own. Your patient may be an 18-year-old daughter with multiple sclerosis, a 25-year-old son who has suffered brain damage in a motorcycle accident, or a 40-year-old spouse whose broken hip mandates long months of physical therapy and daily nursing care. In a nursing home the young adult suffers abnormal and often devastating frustrations and emotional conflicts. His deprivation of youth, family, sex, achievement, a natural social life, and a natural environment add pressure and emphasis to his needs as an individual.

All of us are basically selfish, basically self-centered. It's such an easy matter to think of patients, enlisted men killed in action, victims of fire or automobile accident or other violence, the blind, the poverty-stricken—all the categories of misery that don't directly affect our own lives—as statistics only, not as human beings.

The popular image of both aged and handicapped people denies them the capacity to think and feel. Independence of thought and action, self-assertion, the simple taken-for-granted right of choice are the prerogatives of maturity; yet it is more rare to encounter genuine concern for preserving these birthrights than to meet with compassion for a cat stranded on the limbs of a tree. On the day of admission into a nursing home, these human rights are apt to take flight precipitously.

If it happens that your patient is totally disoriented due to senility, brain damage, or illness, the rights of the individual are still his. He continues to have human feelings and emotions, even if his ability to think and to be self-determining has been damaged or destroyed. Don't make the mistake of confusing these. As long as he lives, he feels; and as long as he feels, whether or not he can express his needs, and whether or not you can identify them, he is nevertheless an individual with human needs and human drives.

I am reminded here of a cherished comment that was spoken to me many years ago. In the nursing home where I was working, a woman ravaged by polio, which she had suffered when she was only fifteen, was in her fortieth year of confinement. She was now in her late 80s; she had become senile, incontinent, and unable to care for her smallest routine needs. Her manner was quiet and sweet. She never intruded herself upon anyone, never asked for help, and never complained. By the same token, nobody took the pains to approach her, perhaps philosophizing to leave well enough alone. I liked her. I responded to her simple acceptance of the fates. Periodically I chatted with her when we met in a corridor or in a dayroom. The briefest sorts of talks, remarking on the shade of blue of the dress she wore or the bright sunshine outside or perhaps the pretty new nurse on the afternoon shift. I made it a habit to hold her hand or smooth her hair, hoping that if she couldn't understand my words, she might be able to understand my touch. She always smiled at me, but never responded in words until one day, to my complete surprise, she said, "You know why I love you? I love you because you treat me like a person, that's why."

A small incident? Very. Yet immeasurable in the significance of what recognition and human warmth can mean to even the most disoriented and the most withdrawn patient. Keep those needs in the forefront of your considerations when you go about selecting a nursing home for your patient.

Before you make the first inquiry, or take the first step toward finding that nursing home, be certain that a nursing home is, in fact, the best solution. I am taking into account the fact that your patient's doctor has referred him to a nursing home, and that his doctor is best qualified to understand the patient's medical condition. But doctors, too, are people—exceptionally busy and pressured people—and sometimes they can be guilty, as all of us are, of speaking in generalities rather than specifics. The doctor may be the first one to acknowledge that there is an equally good answer, perhaps even a better answer, to your patient's need than a nursing home.

Your patient may qualify for a privately—or publicly—administered home-health program (Chapter 2); or perhaps there is a way that *you* can continue his care in your own home or in his. There may be members of the family or close friends who will share the task with you. Depending on the area where you live, perhaps you can call on the Visiting Nurse Service for some professional assistance. Unless your physician specifically prescribes that a registered or licensed practical nurse must be in attendance, you may be able to obtain the services of a man or a woman who is endowed with a warm heart and a strong back. Very often these constitute the only requirements for optimum patient care.

If you can find the way to keep your patient in familiar surroundings, in the midst of his family and friends and neighbors, *without* depriving him of needed professional attention, you will go a long way toward helping him to retain his identity, dignity, and contentment. There may well be practical or psychological obstacles that put this out of the realm of possibility. If it means that other members of your family suffer, if the emotional climate becomes tense, or if you feel resentful, irritable, overfatigued or self-sacrificing, then your patient's illness can easily flare up into a family disability.

In contrast, a good nursing home—one that recognizes human, as well as professional needs—offers many advantages: a wide range of medical and paramedical services, a qualified physician always on call, competent and concerned around-the-clock nursing, rehabilitation therapies, planned recreation programs, professionally supervised diet, and social services. It is possible that a skilled nursing facility may reverse the course of your patient's illness or handicap, and that it may meet his social, as well as his physical, needs. And it can free your patient from the weight of feeling burdensome, indebted, or useless.

Oliver Wendell Holmes once said that "To live is to function." Recovery of natural function from the effects of a number of illnesses, accidents, and disabilities requires twenty-four-hour-a-day professional nursing and regularly administered rehabilitation therapy. In many cases of stroke, for instance, immediate and continued restorative nursing and therapy must be administered by professionals, or full recovery can never be achieved.

It is up to you, to your patient—if he is able—and to his physician to weigh the pro's and con's.

The probe for an honest and optimum answer is difficult, complex, and soul-searching. Tackle it thoroughly and sincerely, for your sake as well as your patient's. Talk it over with the family, who best understand the patient's emotional needs, and certainly with his physician, who best understands his medical needs. Admission into any conscientiously administered health-care facility will require physician referral.

If a nursing home provides the practical and the hopeful answer, make it your business to select the best one you can. May this book help you to find it, and to understand enough of its operation so that your patient—and you—will derive its greatest benefits.

2

The Right Facility for Your Patient

THE MORE YOU KNOW about the product you're shopping for, the more successful you'll be in finding it. First of all, you need to be aware that "nursing home" is a catchall phrase. Although the term has specific definition, its common usage refers to all institutions housing the aged, the ill, or the infirm for a prolonged period of time. In this instance the word "prolonged" is used in its loosest sense, to mean anywhere from a period of weeks to a lifetime. When a layman refers to "a prolonged stay in a nursing home," he may be talking about two weeks or two years in a skilled nursing home, five years in an intermediate care facility, or thirty years in a hospital for chronic disease.

To choose the best facility for *your* patient, you must be aware of his distinctive needs and have a knowledge of the diverse professional programs and personnel available to best fulfill those needs. And you will want an understanding of attendant costs.

If your patient qualifies for Medicare, Medicaid, or both, the matter of cost may be secondary to you. If he is a private patient, there are a number of specific questions you will want answered before a final determination is made.

For the time being, suffice it to say that *Medicare* is an insurance program available for skilled nursing care to almost everyone over 65 years of age and to recipients of social security disability benefits for a minimum period of 24 consecutive months. Benefits in a nursing home are applicable when a patient is enrolled in the Medicare program and meets numerous conditions, including hospitalization within the past 14 days, the same admitting diagnosis that necessitated the hospializa-tion, and medically prescribed daily skilled nursing or rehabilitation care. Although Medicare allows for a maximum period of 100 days per "spell of illness" (specifically defined by the Social Security Administration), the approved number of days in a skilled nursing home is generally considerably less.

Medicaid is an assistance program for the medically indigent of all ages. Contrary to popular belief, most states do not restrict benefits to welfare recipients. They are generally applicable when a patient is financially unable to meet all or part of the cost of nursing-home or other prescribed health care. Medicaid benefits extend for an indefinite period of time or for as long as the patient is both medically and financially qualified.

These benefits, the qualification requirements, and pointers for private-paying patients will be fully discussed in Chapter 7.

However, another aspect of Medicare and Medicaid is pertinent now to your understanding of health-care facilities. Federal standards apply to providers of both programs. The licensed facility that is certified as a provider of Medicare and Medicaid has met federal as well as state standards. The facility that limits its admissions to private-paying patients must be licensed by the state but need not concern itself with federal requirements.

There is wide variance in the licensing standards of individual states. Most states require substantially less by way of professional care and personnel than the federal government. Some states equal or approximate federal requirements. A handful of the more cosmopolitan states are more demanding than the federal government. This is understandable when you look at the problem objectively. For example, New York, with its heavy population and many schools and colleges, has greater resources for providing adequate professional and technical staffing than does the sparsely populated, less sophisticated state.

In selecting the facility for *your* patient, look at only those that have earned federal certification as well as state licensure. Such certification in itself cannot assure you of optimum patient care or personal concern. However, it does mean that the facility has sought and attained federal licensing, and this provides you with at least a basis for assurance.

The range of available health facilities is extensive. The general hospital, which provides the most intensive and consequently the most costly medical care, is not of interest here. The physician has already prescribed a nursing home, so your patient has passed any acute stage of illness.

The only types of hospital that may interest you are a chronic disease or a Veterans Administration hospital. If a chronic disease hospital is located in your immediate neighborhood, or if your patient qualifies for veterans' benefits, you would be wise to discuss the possibility with his physician. If the doctor goes along with such a suggestion, it is probable that your patient will derive needed additional benefits from the more intensive and comprehensive professional programs and personnel available in the hospital setting. Long-term care in a hospital is more costly than in any other type of facility. Well aware of this, the conscientious physician will not approve such institutionalization unless there is a genuine necessity. Medicare and Medicaid benefits are both applicable in the average chronic disease hospital, provided that the patient requires this level of care; veterans' benefits apply, of course, to the Veterans Administration hospital.

Long-Term Care

Nursing Home

The phrase *nursing home* actually refers to two slightly different types of institutions. Although both are responsible for giving the same type of care, the quality and intensity may differ. The *skilled nursing facility* (SNF) is state licensed and also federally certified as a provider of Medicare and Medicaid programs. This means that it has met federal requirements, as well as state. It is equipped to give the intensive nursing care formerly provided by the extended care facility (ECF). The *nursing home* that cannot legally use the adjective "skilled" is state licensed but not federally certified and is, therefore, prohibited from accepting Medicare and Medicaid patients.

Occasionally a woman, generally a nurse, will admit two or three patients into her own residence and call her enterprise a nursing home. Usually this kind of setup is not subject to licensure of any sort and even may be unknown to the licensing agency. I strongly advise against serious consideration of this type of establishment. It *could* provide excellent and personalized nursing; it might have a good physician on call; but it cannot provide the wide range of professional services, personnel, and equipment found in a licensed facility. Further, there is no guarantee that such a home meets any of the licensure requirements for safety, sanitation, dietary supervision, or adequate professional care and observation.

The nursing home that restricts its admission to private-paying patients, and so does not call on reimbursement by federal funds, is subject to state licensing but not federal. This, technically, is the "nursing home" that cannot officially use the qualifying word "skilled." The home may be luxurious in every detail, and costs to patients may run into several thousand dollars a month, but these criteria in no way indicate the quality of professional services. In the few states where standards for licensing equal or exceed federal requirements, it must be assumed that the home prefers to operate without the red tape of government programs. In the many states where licensing criteria are substantially below those demanded for federal certification, it must be wondered whether the nursing home has elected to admit only private patients in order to avoid red tape or whether it has been restricted to private patients because it fails to meet federal standards.

For purposes of brevity, the future use of the term *nursing home* (unless otherwise and specifically indicated) will refer to *licensed skilled nursing facility.*

Licensing. Licensure does not provide you with a guarantee. Obviously a nursing home puts its best foot forward on the day of a licensing survey, and between these annual appointments there can be considerable laxity. It is true, also, that the attitude and thoroughness of licensing agencies and their personnel vary from meticulous to slipshod. This variance often exists in adjacent counties.

The only firm and unequivocal statement that can be made about licensure is that the odds are distinctly in your favor when you know that a nursing home has met state and federal standards and qualifies as a skilled nursing facility. It is a wise move then, when you are on its premises, to ask to see the license of the nursing home and its federal certificate as a provider of Medicare and Medicaid.

Frequently it occurs that a nursing home is granted a provisional license. This means that the facility comes close to meeting all governmental regulations but has a minimal number of deficiencies that are not considered to endanger the health or safety of its patients. In such an instance the nursing home must submit to the licensing agency an acceptable written plan of action for correcting the deficiencies, along with a suitable timetable for full compliance. These revisions must be effected within the allotted time period—frequently the full year is allowed—or permanent licensure is withheld. Obviously your chances of optimum patient care are better if the nursing home's license is *not* provisional.

In order to facilitate your job of selection, you can obtain a listing of all licensed long-term health care facilities in your area (nursing homes and others) by writing or telephoning your state or regional department of health. Simply address the State Department of Health in the capital city of your state (the single exception is Vermont, where the main office is located in Burlington rather than in its capital, Montpelier). Such a listing will not indicate whether or not the home's license is conditional, so it is wise to see this for yourself.

Many nursing homes are approved by the Joint Commission for Accreditation of Hospitals and proudly display this certificate. The standards of the Joint Commission are notoriously and uniformly both excellent and comprehensive. Its certificate of accreditation implies that the highest standards have been met; but here, again, such accreditation covers a considerable period—in this case, two years—and between surveys there is no means of ascertaining that these criteria are continuously met. In spite of this, accreditation by the Joint Commission, while not essential, serves to give you further assurance of the home's standing.

Skilled Nursing Facility (SNF)

The most inclusive and intensive professional care, after the hospital, is provided by the skilled nursing facility. These facilities provide medical care, around-the-clock nursing, recreation, social services, professional dietary supervision, diagnostic X-ray, laboratory, and pharmaceutical services, dental care, and usually podiatry, optometry, physical therapy, occupational therapy, speech therapy, and audiology. If any of these services is not available at the nursing home, it is customary for arrangements to be made to use the services of a nearby hospital or other health facility. If, however, a nursing home has no occupational therapy, for instance, and no arrangements to supply it, the home is forbidden by law to accept a patient whose physician has prescribed this form of therapy for him. The details of the SNF programs are discussed later.

Admissions. Admission to a skilled nursing facility requires a medical prescription for skilled nursing or professional rehabilitation care. The physician provides the nursing home with the patient's current medical findings and diagnoses, along with his medical history and his potential for rehabilitation.

Some states restrict admission to patients 21 years of age or older; in others there is no age limit. Most states restrict admissions to patients suffering physical impairment, not psychiatric. In the case of the senile patient, senility is a physical disorder based on hardening of the arteries of the brain (cerebral arteriosclerosis). Although its manifestations frequently parallel psychoses, the senile patient is freely admitted to the nursing home since his illness is classified as vascular rather than mental. Skilled nursing facilities often accept patients transferred from mental hospitals with diagnoses of "burned out" psychoses. This means that a patient once confined to a mental hospital for schizophrenia or severe depression, for instance, has progressed beyond the need for psychiatric treatment. He has now achieved a plateau where he is harmless to himself and to others but is incapable of being restored to independence in the activities of daily living or in the resumption of self-reliance.

Occasionally nursing homes send either a social worker or a member of the nursing staff for a pre-admission interview with the prospective patient and members of his family.

Administration. Skilled nursing homes are required t. have full-time administrators. Nursing-home administrators must be licensed by the state's licensing agency. Licenses are based on combinations of experience, education, written examination, and compulsory state approved continuing education, and must be renewed at one- or two-year intervals, depending on the state. Assistant administrators must meet the same requirements, but states vary in their determination of the numbers of beds in a nursing home that necessitate an assistant director.

Medical Care. Continuing physician service has always been a mandate of the federal government. The post of medical director has been required by many individual states, but only in December 1974 did it become a federal requirement, with an allowance of one full year from that date to fill the position. The services of a competent medical director are of utmost value in achieving optimum patient care. In the absence of a medical director, an *advisory physician* has assisted the administrator in establishing and enforcing medical policies. In certain rural areas where it may not be possible to secure a medical director, the SNF will be permitted to continue operation with the services of an advisory physician.

The role of the medical director is pertinent and comprehensive. He determines all medical and medical-related policies, provides for full-time coverage for emergencies, supervises medical and paramedical services, and performs numerous salient duties as described in Chapter 4.

Unless the nursing home is so small that one physician can provide competent care to all its patients, then there is a staff of general practitioners and internists who care for individual patients. A staff of consultant physicians covers such specialties as cardiology, urology, ophthalmology, orthopedics, neurology, psychiatry, and others.

Nursing. Members of nursing staff play a vital role, since it is their primary responsibility to fulfill physicians' orders. As in hospitals, physicians are accountable for the medical progress of their patients. However, barring emergencies, medical visits are on a monthly basis (sometimes bimonthly after ninety days) rather than daily (Chapter 4). Although doctors are always on call for emergencies and for instructions, prescriptions, and advice, they are not on the premises daily, and nurses, therefore, shoulder a greater responsibility for patients in a nursing home than in a hospital.

Contrary to the hospital situation, the majority of nursing personnel is comprised of unlicensed aides and orderlies who report directly to licensed nurses. Federal regulations call for licensed staff nurses and licensed charge nurses around the clock (these can be registered or practical nurses) but require only one registered staff nurse who must be assigned to day tours seven days a week. (Occasionally, under stringent circumstances, this requirement is lowered to five days a week.) In addition, the staff must include a full-time nursing director, qualified as a registered nurse, who is responsible for the overall training and the operation and performance of the entire nursing staff. The nursing director may serve also as day-tour charge nurse if the number of patients is limited to sixty. If patient population exceeds this figure, then an additional registered or practical nurse is assigned this task.

Larger skilled nursing facilities, located in states with higher requirements, call for licensed staff nurses, charge nurses, and unless the number of patients is extremely small, nursing supervisors. Registered nurses serve as assistant director of nursing (depending on the size of the home) and often as in-service education director. The positions of nursing director, assistant director, and in-service education director can be filled by one or two nurses rather than three.

Licensed nurses are responsible for skilled nursing care such as intravenous feedings, postoperative colostomy or tracheotomy care, administration of oral, intramuscular, and intravenous medications, suctioning, and constant professional observation to include the early detection of change in a patient's condition that may require the physician's immediate attention and prescribed treatment. These represent only a few of the duties classified as *skilled* nursing care.

Services such as bed-making, bed baths, bedpans, personal grooming, assistance with eating or walking, and other equally important but less skilled functions are carried out by aides and orderlies who are unlicensed. These aides and orderlies, however, usually spend more time and have more direct contact with your patient than the licensed personnel. Their roles must not be underestimated. On the contrary, these employees are to be highly respected for the difficult and often dreary tasks they perform and for their continuous contribution to your patient's daily comfort and well-being.

Transfer Agreements. The skilled nursing facility is almost always affiliated with a nearby general hospital to provide for emergency treatment or admission of patients and for the use of hospital personnel and portable equipment in the nursing home should they be indicated. These affiliations are referred to as "transfer agreements" and are actually written contracts. The nursing home is apt to have affiliation, too, with one or more facilities rendering *less* specialized care so that as a patient progresses in health status and in self-maintenance he can be transferred to a less costly institution that allows him increased independence and a program geared more to social than to medical and nursing needs.

It is completely appropriate for you to inquire at the nursing home as to what transfer agreements it may have. The hospital affiliation should be of special importance to you, since your patient could be transferred there within minutes of an emergent or critical turn in his condition. Since time is not crucial in transferring a patient to a facility offering less specialized care, the physician or, in his absence, a designated staff member of the nursing home is obligated to discuss the move with your patient (if possible) and with you before any action is taken.

Costs. The cost of care in a skilled nursing facility varies. Although it is high, it is considerably less than in the hospital. Nursing home care is less intensive; equipment is less varied, less sophisticated, and less expensive than the hospital's; the ratio of nursing-home personnel to patients is one to one, or less, while in the hospital it is approximately three and a half to one; and—except for a rare and noteworthy exception—the nursing home does not carry the costly burdens of research, teaching, and clinic services.

Nursing homes, like hospitals, are private (profit-making), voluntary (nonprofit), or government financed. Although most hospitals are voluntary, most nursing homes are private and are operated for profit. Comparatively few (approximately 10 percent) are voluntary. Government nursing homes (about 5 percent) exist usually on the local level. However, government funding on federal, state, and frequently on county levels is accountable for costs of the Medicaid program, and the federal government is solely responsible for Medicare payments as well as all Veterans Administration institutions.

Intermediate Care Facility (ICF)

Sometimes referred to as a health related facility, the intermediate care facility offers substantially less by way of professional staffing and services than the skilled nursing home. Its goal is to tend patients who require a minimal level of health related care. Services are geared to meet the patient's social, dietary, and routine daily needs and activities rather than the medical, nursing, and rehabilitation objectives of the skilled nursing facility.

Admissions. The only requirement for admission is that the patient's needs must be of such a nature that they can be met by the ICF and those community resources with which it is affiliated. No further restrictions are identified. (Some intermediate care facilities are geared to the exclusive care of mental retardation, in which case programs and personnel are subject to special pertinent qualifications. This type of facility is not included in our present discussion, since the focus here is on physical impairment.)

Administration. A full-time administrator, state-licensed as a nursing-home administrator, is required.

Medical Care. Each patient is under the continuing supervision of a physician "as needed." Medical visits are routinely scheduled at sixty-day intervals; however, if the attending physician justifies and documents in writing that the patient requires less frequent medical visits, the sixty-day provision can be amended accordingly. Complete physical examinations are conducted at least annually. All medications are reviewed quarterly by the attending physician or staff doctor and on a monthly basis by a registered nurse. Emergency medical care is always available.

Nursing. The approved intermediate care facility has at least one licensed nurse assigned to the day shift seven days a week as supervisor of health services. If she is a practical nurse, then a registered nurse serves as her supervisor and consultant at regular intervals of as little as four hours weekly. A nursing *director* is not required. The charge "nurse" need be neither a registered nor a practical nurse but must be approved as having met other specific educational criteria required by the state.

Aides assist patients in the activities of daily living, a focal point in the goals of the intermediate care facility. These activities include grooming, walking, eating, toileting, and other aspects of personal care. It is one of the primary objectives of intermediate care to restore the patient to the greatest level of independence in the activities of daily living (ADL) of which he is capable. Written care plans are developed for all patients, and these are reevaluated at regular intervals and revised when indicated.

Other Services and Policies. The intermediate care facility provides an organized recreation program, communal dining room, rehabilitation services either on the premises or available through outside resources, isolation rooms and isolation techniques in case of infectious disease, accurate maintenance of medical records and their storage for a minimum period of three years, written and rehearsed fire and disaster plans, written personnel policies and procedures, orientation and in-service education programs for the staff, professionally established policies for the storage, disposal, and records of drugs, and provision for dental services. All services are rendered on an "as needed" basis.

Although these programs and policies parallel many of those incorporated in the skilled nursing facility, they are provided on a less intensive basis, and standards for professional staffing and consultation are less exacting. Many professionals are approved by either training *or* experience, rather than the combination of the two that is demanded by the skilled nursing facility. A number of requirements, including fire inspection reports, laundry facilities, and areas for food preparation, recreation, and dayrooms, have been eliminated.

Transfer Agreements. As with the skilled nursing home, the intermediate care facility usually has a transfer agreement with a neighborhood general hospital and also may have a transfer agreement with one or more skilled nursing homes. In this way a patient whose condition changes so that he requires more intensive care can be transferred to either a hospital or a nursing home according to the physician's judgment. Except for emergency transfer to a hospital, relatives are contacted before the patient is discharged.

Costs. The cost of care in an intermediate facility, as with the level of care, is less than in a skilled nursing facility. Medicare reimbursement is never applicable because skilled nursing is available on a token basis only, and the medical conditions of patients have progressed beyond the rigid requirements necessary for eligibility. Patients who qualify for Medicaid are entitled to these benefits when the facility meets federal standards. ICF's are state licensed, and some are certified by the federal government as providers of Medicaid assistance.

On occasion, one home or one building is divided into areas to accommodate patients requiring skilled nursing and patients requiring intermediate care services. In these circumstances, staffing, programming, and costs vary in direct proportion to the intensity and range of services provided.

Home Health Programs

Almost invariably hospital-based, home health programs provide a variety of services to the patient in his home. According to the physician's orders, these can include the part-time services of licensed nurses or of nursing aides. They can provide physical, occupational, and speech therapies; medical social services; and some medical supplies, as well as training and supervision in the use of medical appliances. These programs are covered by Part B of Medicare (Chapter 7), provided that the agency is Medicare approved, and provided that the patient has been in a hospital or skilled nursing facility within the past fourteen days and his physician certifies that home health visits are medically essential and for the same condition that initially hospitalized him.

Part B of Medicare will pay the full cost of one hundred home health visits during each benefit period. However, coverage does not necessarily extend for one hundred days, since a nurse and a therapist might well visit the patient during the same afternoon. Medicaid meets these costs when the patient is medically indigent and either does not have Medicare coverage or needs financial assistance in meeting the deductible billing.

Day Hospitals

Mostly a gleam in the eye of the professional health-care planner, only a handful of day hospitals are now in operation. These programs are usually a part of existing general hospitals or hospital complexes and provide the care indicated by their name: highly skilled medical, paramedical, nursing, social, and rehabilitation services administered during the daytime hours when the patient is on the premises.

The concept allows for the best of two possible worlds for those patients who do *not* require twenty-four-hour a day skilled nursing care or observation. The day hospital offers medically prescribed skilled professional care during an eight-hour day (sometimes less, depending on the patient's need), up to five days a week, while at the same time allowing him to be at home with his family evenings and weekends. Emphasis is usually on rehabilitation designed to meet the physical and emotional needs of the patient. Members of the family are trained to provide personal care for the patient during the hours he is away from the day hospital, and are also professionally guided to an understanding and acceptance of their own emotional needs as well as the patient's. In all instances the patient's attending physician retains medical management. Transportation, as a rule, is up to the patient or his family, but in some instances it is provided by the day hospital.

These facilities are state licensed and certified as providers of Medicaid when they meet federal standards. Although Part A of Medicare is not applicable, since services are not continuous and patients do not require constant professional care, Part B will absorb at least some of the costs.

It must be emphasized that the day hospital is rare, and the chance of finding one anywhere near you is highly improbable. The day hospital is not to be confused with the *day care center*, which is geared more to social activity than to professional health services.

Out-Patient Services

Your patient's needs might be met by the out-patient services in a hospital. Only his physician can determine this. Most voluntary general hospitals have out-patient clinics geared to give the patient medical, technical, and therapeutic services, *but not on a continuing basis* as given to the in-patient. Also, there is the unwieldy and often impractical or insoluble problem of transporting your patient back and forth from the hospital, generally for one- or two-hour sessions, on a daily or near daily basis. Medicare (Part B) and Medicaid programs can provide coverage for hospital out-patient services when they are prescribed by the physician.

Other Classifications

Other long-term health-care facilities include the rehabilitation center (usually a skilled nursing facility that emphasizes rehabilitation programs), convalescent home, comprehensive care facility, intensive nursing care facility and the personal care home. These are usually either skilled nursing facilities, nursing homes or intermediate care facilities. You must inquire as to the exact services rendered. The information here should enable you to place that facility in one of these classifications.

Perhaps, in a way, this chapter can be likened to the yellow pages of the telephone book, where "your fingers do the walking"—at least some of the walking. Hopefully you will now have a better understanding of the type of care most appropriate for your patient.

It should be emphasized with all vigor and intensity that if your patient is disoriented, it is expedient for you to look for a facility that caters to disoriented patients, where the staff will be familiar and empathetic with your patient's emotional, recreational, and social needs, as well as his medical ones. If your patient is physically handicapped, find a nursing center that specializes in rehabilitation; if he needs speech therapy, be sure that there is a daily—or near daily—professional program. If your patient is young, don't let him be the only young patient or one of just a handful; find the facility that serves numerous young patients and caters to *their* emotional, recreational, and social needs. If your patient is a child, you may be fortunate in finding a pediatric nursing home. If your patient is a brain-damaged adolescent, there are a few facilities geared to meet these special needs.

Certainly it is improbable, if not impossible, that any one long-term facility, skilled nursing home or other, can meet the special and equally fundamental needs of all the categories of patients who require long-term care. It behooves you to play demigod in the awesome task before you: the determination of the *one* facility best suited to fill the myriad needs of the patient you have elected to help.

Granted, there may or may not be time to do this "shopping" at the outset. Your patient's physician may transfer him to a home within a few days after he first suggests it. And his choice of nursing home or other health-care facility may be a fortuitous one, with no need for you to ever look elsewhere. On the other hand, you may have a few weeks or many weeks to plan the best possible placement for your patient; or you and your patient may be unhappy with the doctor's selection and, after a while, agree to make a change.

It has been assumed that the facility you are looking for is a nursing home. Is it still a nursing home? One that is licensed as a skilled nursing facility? Then, with time, effort, and know-how, you can accomplish wonders in seeking out the home that will bring your patient good care, respect, and a measure of contentment.

The following guidelines will help you in your search.

3

The Physical Plant

THE ONE THING you may know of the nursing home in advance of your visit (other than licensure) is its reputation—but don't put too much faith in that. It is of negative value, at best. If the home has a poor reputation, you probably won't take the time to go to see it, and the chances are that the poor reputation is warranted. On the reverse, however, a good reputation, one that would direct you to a nursing home's doorsteps, is not necessarily merited.

One of the biggest and best-known nursing homes in the country enjoys a superb reputation. But that esteem is held by the general public, not by its patients or their families. The nursing home hires a well-experienced publicity man. Also, it is a member organization of one of the largest and wealthiest federated charities in the nation, and the federation has a well-staffed, well-paid public relations department. The nursing home boasts a full gamut of services and professional and paraprofessional personnel. Most of the departments—and the personnel—are excellent, but the most important area of all, the nursing department, is so deficient in conscience and concern, so lacking in recognition of the patient as an individual, that despite the glowing reputation of the nursing home, it houses the unhappiest patients I have ever known.

This inability to recognize the *person* within the patient is shared, even fostered, by the administrator who otherwise would not tolerate the attitude of members of the nursing staff. Yet the administrator exudes charm and an air of sincerity and warmth. Were you to meet with him, take his word and the home's reputation at face value, you would be sure that you had made the best possible selection for your patient. Conversely, were you to spend an hour or two in the nursing areas and the corridors, you would observe the unanswered calls of totally dependent patients, the harsh tones used by the nursing staff in addressing patients, and the pervading aura of indifference. This exemplifies another reason why you are urged to do your own shopping and conduct your own investigation.

Neighborhood, Building, Grounds. Your first direct experience with any nursing home is the neighborhood, the building itself, and the grounds. Hopefully, you will be able to choose a location that is readily accessible to you and to other family members and friends of your patient. Remember that he hasn't changed his basic needs as an individual, except that those needs are accentuated by his placement in an unnatural environment. Now, more than ever before, he will need the security of having loved ones near him as frequently as possible, of feeling remembered and loved, and of still being a member of the family, as well as a member of society.

Aside from a well-groomed appearance, it is totally unimportant whether or not the building and grounds are breathtakingly beautiful or utterly ordinary. It *is* important that there are grounds or patios suitable and accessible to the patients for their enjoyment in the warm weather. Ramps may be essential for patients using wheelchairs, crutches, or walkers.

The same principle applies to the interior of the building. An attractive décor is pleasant and reassuring but of no real value. The building itself must be safe, comfortable, and spacious. Handsome drapes, exquisitely detailed chairs and end tables, frescoes on lobby walls, will add nothing to your patient's comfort, happiness, or health. How soon they will fade into the background, and he will cease to notice them at all!

Safety measures. The single most important factor about the building is safety. You will, of course, want a building of fire-resistive construction (not wood frame) and assurance that all safety measures pertaining to fire prevention and control are in effect. Many factors are involved, some of them dependent on the size of the building and whether or not it is multiple-storied. The following factors are vital: stairways enclosed and located functionally at key points; an adequate number of elevators; automatic sprinkler systems in critical areas; fire doors; and fire alarms and fire-fighting equipment located strategically throughout the building, along with posted notices, printed clearly and succinctly, listing the steps to be taken in case of fire. You will want to know whether or not there is a written emergency evacuation plan and whether routine fire drills are held on all shifts.

All of these safety items should be in order in the licensed nursing home. Unfortunately, however, a recent fifteen-state survey conducted by the Department of Health, Education and Welfare showed that inadequate fire safety was one of the most frequent deficiencies found in nursing homes. So much always depends on the discerning eye of the individual or the team responsible for licensing. For example, Mr. Smith is charged with determining safety measures and all factors pertaining to sanitation, emergency equipment, and other physical aspects of the building. He may be a whiz at his job and scrutinize every detail. He may find everything in order, or he may demand that it be put in order without delay. On the other hand, he may be less exacting; or perhaps he's had an argument with his wife on the morning of the survey, or his best suit has been lost by the dry cleaner, and he's not as perceptive or as astute as usual.

You may well want to conduct your own investigation. Start with a telephone call or a visit to the local fire department which will answer most of your questions. Then take your own tour of the building to observe equipment; talk with the administrator about sprinkler systems and emergency evacuation plans; and talk with a number of patients about the frequency and effectiveness of fire drills.

Many nursing homes have safety committees comprised of representatives of all departments. These committees usually meet on a monthly basis and are responsible for promoting safety awareness and safety measures for both the patients and the personnel. Surely the existence of such a committee adds to the safety of the building and its patients. Whoever interviews you when you visit the nursing home will be in a position to tell you whether or not such a committee exists. An *actively* functioning safety committee offers the advantages of safety-minded personnel with regularly scheduled opportunities to air and exchange their ideas. In addition, it is indicative of a people-oriented administration.

The effectiveness of the call-bell system, one of the most urgent safety factors in any nursing home, will require a little discernment on your part. In hospitals every patient has a call-bell at his bedside for summoning the assistance of a nurse. This is true for the nursing-home patient as well. But call-bells are installed in different ways.

In every instance, a panel of lights at the nursing station identifies the location of the bed where the patient is ringing for help. A buzzer should, and generally does, accompany the light. Frequently this call-bell panel is located on a wall behind the desk where nurses sit and work and often use the telephone. The two aspects of this system most important for your patient's safety as well as his convenience are first, Is there a buzzer? And is the buzzer loud enough to attract the nurse's attention if she is engaged in a conversation or if her back is turned to the panel and the light that locates the patient's bed? Does the buzzer sound just once or does it continue to signal? Second, many such systems are set up so that the nurse can disconnect the signal through a switch on the panel itself. This is totally inadequate. Although most nurses are conscientious and concerned, significant numbers are more interested in their own tired feet and the pressures of the day's work. It is essential to your patient that the signal can be turned off *at his bedside only.* This is the modern and the single effective way of being certain that a nurse will come to the aid of the patient when he calls.

There is an added and obvious advantage if your patient's room is located where it can be viewed from the nursing station. However, this is not essential if the call-bell system is effective and the nursing staff is conscientious.

Maintenance. Although safety is your number one concern about the building, it is not the sum and substance of all that you want. Look for both cleanliness and good maintenance as well as adequate furnishings and equipment. Be on the lookout for insects or rodents, especially in areas adjacent to the kitchen, garbage disposal, and soiled laundry storage. Notice if all entrances are protected by screen doors during warm weather.

Be aware of odor. Optimally, there should be none. A strong scent of urine (not to be confused with ammonia) is indicative of poor nursing, poor housekeeping, or both. A heavy aroma of perfumed spray is generally indicative of an effort to mask these same deficiencies.

Carpeting is being used more and more frequently in modern nursing homes. Its effect is pleasant to the eye, but it can constitute a serious deterrent to sanitation, since all nursing homes care for a substantial number of incontinent patients and, further, there is always accidental spillage of foods, medications, and other items that deposit dirt and stain. Tiling is infinitely easier to keep scrupulously clean. The only advantage to carpeting for your patient is if he is ambulatory, yet unsteady on his feet, or dependent on crutches or a walker. Then carpeting will give him additional security in walking. It will not only prevent slipping, but it will lend psychological support that can be fundamental to improving his ambulation. Imagine learning to maneuver with crutches, conscious of pain in a broken hip or a ruptured disc, and looking ahead down a long corridor of freshly waxed shining tiles. If your patient is wheelchair-bound, however, then tiling will facilitate his handling of the wheelchair, while carpeting will impede it.

Space. Look also for adequate space, comfort, and convenience. Space is meaningful only as it affects the patients. In the corridors, look for width that allows easy passage of two patients using wheelchairs, crutches, or walkers. Strong, substantial handrails spell out security and safety for the many patients who rely on them; and they are indications of the thought and the financing that went into planning a building for the welfare of the patients. Slim handrails that resemble (or may be) closet poles can be inadequate, both physically and psychologically.

An adequate number of drinking fountains (with easily accessible paper cups) should be located along the corridors, as should an adequate number of public telephones. Because of the large number of wheelchair patients, telephone booths are impractical; instead, Plexiglas panels at the sides of the phones allow at least a modicum of privacy, and there should be ledges beneath the phones for paper and pen. The telephones should be installed at heights convenient for wheelchair patients and for those who are able to stand.

Space is a vital factor for privacy, social activities, and comfort. It's impractical to expect a nursing home to provide enough space to guarantee patients privacy with all their visitors (aside from one-bedded rooms). However, the more space that is devoted to dayrooms, library, dining room, patio, and grounds, the better the chances are of finding a nook for private conversation with family or friends.

One or more dining rooms allow mealtimes to be congenial get-togethers, an opportunity denied patients who are restricted to eating in their bedrooms.

A canteen adds immeasurably to patient comfort by supplying not only coffee, soda, cigarettes, and snacks, but also by making available to patients cosmetics, combs and brushes, stockings and socks, and other small items of personal need. However, a word of caution: take note of the prices. Some nursing homes use these shops as a means of making inordinate profit.

Recreation should be allotted a large room of its own and should be encouraged to spill over into the dining room, dayroom, and other areas so that, with the help of volunteers, programs can be held concurrently for groups with differing interests and differing capabilities. A small nursing home may have to confine recreation programs to the dining room and possibly the dayroom. If the home does not have a chapel, then religious services are likely to be held in the recreation room, dining room, or dayroom.

A patient-planned nursing home has a library with a wide selection of well-kept books and current magazines readily accessible to all patients. In addition, if the recreation room is closed to patients on weekends and evenings, the library is the logical area for an assortment of games such as chess, checkers, Monopoly, Scrabble, picture puzzles, crossword puzzles, playing cards, and other pastimes that the patients can enjoy on their own. The library should be open at all times. If lack of space prohibits a library, books and games can be housed in dayrooms.

Physical therapy and occupational therapy quarters are essential to you only if either has been prescribed for your patient. Details of equipment to look for will be covered in Chapter 6. Speech therapy and audiology may or may not have their own quarters, but this is of no major consequence, since these can be administered in any area that affords a measure of privacy or at the patient's bedside.

Rooms should be allotted for medical examination (patient treatment rooms) and also for isolation in the event that a patient develops a contagious disease. An isolation room is a requirement of federal law and must be equipped with its own hand-washing and toilet facilities.

Service Areas. The kitchen is important to you as an indication of cleanliness and sanitary standards. A dishwashing machine is of utmost importance toward ensuring both. Areas for food preparation, dishwashing, and garbage must be separated. (Dietary services will be covered in Chapter 5.)

The only items of kitchen *equipment* that need to concern you (aside from the dishwasher) are the carts that transport food to the dining rooms and patients' floors. The carts should be closed for hygienic purposes; and if not, how are plates of food covered, and how are foods protected from contamination once they leave the kitchen? Likewise, some food carts are heated. If they are, you will want to ascertain that cold foods are transported separately. If they are not, you will want to know how foods are kept hot going from the kitchen. Frequently hot pellets are used, and these are placed in rounded metal bowls that support china or plastic plates.

A growing number of nursing homes use "convenience foods" (actually, frozen meals that require only heating) and disposable plates and utensils. Ask yourself if you would elect to eat prepared frozen meals three times a day every day of the week, and how you would enjoy those meals eaten from paper plates with plastic tableware. This kind of makeshift eating is fine on occasion, when all the family is rushing to prepare for an evening out or if guests are expected shortly after the dinner hour, but it is extremely doubtful that anyone would choose this sort of fare or service on a regular basis. Ever eat a soft-boiled egg from a cardboard bowl with a plastic spoon? In a nursing home, meals become focal points of the day. No matter how important or unimportant the matter of eating has been to your patient in the past, unless his illness has destroyed his appetite entirely, he will want more enjoyment from his meals than he ever did before.

A beauty parlor and a barbershop (or one room to accommodate both) meet not only the need for the patient's good grooming, but also his need for self-respect in self-imagery. Shaving is usually performed at the patient's bedside by a member of the nursing staff, but shampoos and haircuts for men must be provided on a regular basis, as well as shampoos, haircuts, hair-sets, and even permanent waves for women.

A storage room for patients' belongings is a rare and wonderful thing to find. Under the stress of today's economy it is doubtful that you will find it, so it is not a must. But if you are lucky enough to stumble across a nursing home that furnishes space for patients' out-of-season clothing and for personal possessions that have a sentimental or other special meaning to them, then chances are that you have found a nursing home that does, indeed, care about its patients as individuals with personal needs.

Although a nursing home may choose to rent its linens, or use a professional laundry for their upkeep, it is also responsible for patients' personal laundry, such as underwear, sleepwear, washable dresses, shirts and slacks, stockings and socks. In most states this is a mandatory service to be performed *without charge to the patient.* Therefore, you will want to see for yourself what laundry equipment is on the premises and what schedule is in effect to guarantee this service at regular and frequent intervals. Dry cleaning is sent out by the nursing home and billed to the patient.

Equipment. Air conditioning is another manifestation of concern. Every nursing home supplies heat for cold weather, but don't assume that it offers air conditioning for hot weather. A number of homes that were built many years ago are not electrically equipped to provide this comfort. Some administrators of newly constructed nursing homes claim that a few illnesses respond poorly to cold air, and, therefore, air conditioning is limited to the lobby and offices. Your patient's physician is the only one who can give you the right advice on this particular subject. Chances are that cool air will do your patient a great deal more good than harm. The best arrangement is a combination heating and cooling appliance installed in each patient's room with its own individual thermostat. Central air conditioning is satisfactory, as is the individual air conditioning unit installed in a window or under a window of every room.

However, do not take anything for granted. From the outside of one modern nursing home that opened in the fall of the year, as well as within, it was immediately apparent that under every window was positioned an air conditioning sleeve clearly and boldly identified with the name of a leading air conditioner manufacturer. Every relative who admitted a patient assumed that with the advent of hot weather air conditioners would be installed in those sleeves. Everyone who made this assumption was wrong. The appliances were installed for the comfort (and consequently the greater work output) of personnel, but not for the patients. When relatives inquired, they were told that the installation of an air conditioner would be at their own expense. Not only did this prove to be a financial hardship for many patients, and a total impossibility for others, it also frequently presented an untenable position for patients in a two- or four-bedded room where one suffered from the heat, while another disliked cold forced air, or would not or could not share the cost. So when you are escorted through the nursing home on your initial visit, inquire about air conditioning. It might be wise, too, to ask a few of the patients.

Hot water (one temperature for patient use and a much higher degree for dishwashing and laundry); emergency equipment to ensure water and electric power in critical areas; adequate lighting, heating, and ventilation; and limitation of

sound are all regulated by the federal government and constitute conditions for federal certification.

Some nursing homes offer bedrooms with double exposure
(rare), and some are wise enough to place beds on adjacent
walls so that two patients can look directly into each other's
faces, and conversation and eye contact are both facilitated.
Under the usual arrangement of beds placed side by side, visual
contact is eye to navel. Whatever the placement of beds, there
must be cubicle curtains of fireproof fabric (or the equivalent)
that allow complete privacy for each patient, and the room
must be spacious enough to permit the easy use of wheelchairs.
Federal and state codes specify actual room size and the space
required around each bed, as well as the requirement that
all bedrooms have outside windows, and doors opening onto
corridors.

Electric beds offer a wonderful convenience to patients, allowing them to raise or lower their mattresses by the touch of a
lever. Chances are that you won't find these, and there are two
reasons for their scarcity: one, they are almost prohibitively expensive; and, two, many patients suffer from illnesses that require a raised bed or, perhaps, a flat bed, and it is therefore
medically sound to limit the raising or lowering of the mattress
to the nursing staff.

There will be chairs in the room, but are they comfortable
upholstered armchairs in which your patient can relax? Are
they sturdily built so they won't tip over? And is there adequate lighting adjacent to the chair, as well as to the bed, so he
can read or write with comfort and ease? Is there a small table
or a wide arm to the chair that will allow him to rest his book
or write letters?

Are drawer space and closet space adequate? Don't expect
either to measure up to what he has at home. It won't. By "adequate" I mean exactly that, and no more. Will it suffice for the
comparatively few belongings he will keep with him during his
nursing-home stay? Is there a sink in the room for washing, a

mirror, racks for towels, a bedside table with a few drawers for those belongings that he may want to reach from his bed?

Federal requirements call for "adequate" bath and toilet facilities, but state codes are apt to be more specific. Some homes go beyond the minimum requirements. More important, are there grab bars and call-bells adjacent to each toilet and tub or shower? And is space adequate to allow for wheelchair patients and attendants? Find out for yourself how many patients must share toilet facilities with yours, and how many showers or bathtubs are located on his floor. Just as rare good fortune alone will lead you to the nursing home that offers double exposure in the patients' bedrooms, so might this same good fortune lead you to the occasional nursing home that offers full bathroom facilities to every two or four patients.

Television can help to pass many lonely hours, but don't be too quickly impressed if you find a set in every patient's room. One of the finest nursing homes I have ever known made it a policy to require written medical approval for a patient to have a TV set in his bedroom. The reasoning? Both simple and wise. The motivation to watch television became instrumental in getting a patient up out of bed, out of his room, and into the dayroom where two large colored television sets were installed, one at either end of the room. This provided the patient with mild exercise by way of getting to and from the dayroom and also with the companionship of other patients watching television or simply socializing among themselves.

You will look for other things in the physical plant: equipment or built-in conveniences that have particular meaning to you or your patient. The items covered here are limited to those that are probably important to everyone. Almost without exception these are aspects that you can see and determine for yourself. Just be sure that you know how to look at what you see.

4

Yardsticks: Administrative and Medical

THE TOTAL CARE of the patient—his physical, emotional, and social well-being—is the primary goal of any good nursing home. It must be the focal point of policies developed through the joint efforts of the owners or trustees, the administrator, and the medical director or advisory physician. These policies should be adapted to meet the full range of the patient's needs and, when possible, his preferences. In contrast to the hospital, where patients must conform to rigid schedules because of the pressure of time and the multiplicity of services and personnel involved, the nursing home must take into account the projected length of the patient's stay and his need for a relaxed and homelike atmosphere.

It is with the idea of emphasizing this homelike atmosphere that many nursing homes make it a practice to refer to the patient as a resident. I used to agree with this theory until an incident happened to me that completely changed my viewpoint.

About seven or eight years ago I was hospitalized for a number of weeks, in traction because of a back injury. A close friend of mine, the head of the social service department in a large nursing home, called me on the phone and said, "Well, I hear you're a resident now." Without thinking, I veritably snapped at her, "*Don't* call me a resident! I'm a patient." Suddenly I had realized that the word "resident" has a sound of forever to it, but that the word "patient" has a temporary connotation, and therefore brings with it the valuable ingredient of hope. From that time on I have referred only to "patients."

Each staff member has his own area of assignment. He must adhere to the specifications of his written job description, abide by all established rules, regulations, and policies of the home, and respect the patient as an individual endowed with inherent and inalienable human rights. The objectives of the nursing home can be met only if all personnel work together as a team. Each employee's job is essential to the whole; for the whole, as all of us learned back in grammar school, is but the sum of its parts.

The organizational chart which follows is typical for all nursing homes. It will give you an understanding of lines of authority and the knowledge of where to bring questions or complaints, if necessary, after your patient is admitted. If your problem relates to nursing, for instance, speak first to the aide or staff nurse who attends your patient. If you are unhappy with the response, then go to the head nurse. If you remain dissatisfied, next in line is the nursing supervisor, then the nursing director, and last in line, the administrator. The sole reason for omitting the medical director (or advisory physician) is its impracticability. He is not always available, while the administrator generally is. Further, the nursing home and its problems constitute a relatively small part of the medical director's overall time and effort, whereas they remain the full concern of the administrator, who is likely to have a more comprehensive understanding of the total picture. (If the problem is a major one, then, failing all else, you are free to contact the local or state department of health, your local

TYPICAL ORGANIZATIONAL CHART

Solid lines indicate "reports to"; dotted lines indicate "works in conjunction with."

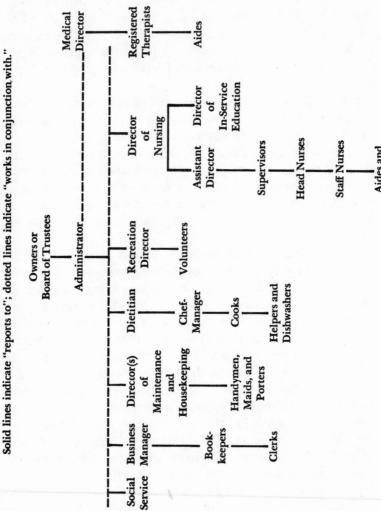

social security or social services office, or your congressman or senator.)

It is not only customary to follow such procedure, but other tactics can create chaos and almost certainly result in hard feelings toward you. As an example: if an aide or a staff nurse commits an error in judgment; if she thoughtlessly offends or inconveniences or even angers your patient, she may well be resentful if he reports the incident to the nursing director or the administrator, and this resentment is apt to show itself in her attitude toward your patient. On the other hand, if she is approached directly and is given the opportunity to handle the matter on a one-to-one basis, and to relieve the problem before it mushrooms, then the likelihood is excellent that she will resume a comfortable relationship with your patient, and he with her.

The objective of the delegation of authority is the support of those who directly serve the patients. Authority to act is delegated from the owners through the administrator and the department heads to every person working in the institution.

The Administrator

The obligation of the nursing home and its administrator is the provision of a full range of high quality professional and paraprofessional patient services and an atmosphere of warmth, reassurance, respect, and encouragement to patients as well as to their relatives and friends.

The owners or trustees of the nursing home have the prerogative of establishing the policies of the facility, within accepted guidelines. Although the administrator works along with them and may exert a strong influence on both practical and ideological planning, his basic function is to enforce the policies as they are adopted by the governing body. It is evident that an administrator who views the welfare of the patients as his primary responsibility cannot share viewpoints or effectively administer policies that negate the patients' well-being.

The administrator shoulders full responsibility for achieving the goals of the home and must guide, supervise, and work closely with all his department heads toward this common objective. He must ascertain that his departments always meet all federal, state, and local government regulations pertaining to nursing homes and all laws protecting patients and staff. These laws include and enforce admission of patients without regard to race, color, or national origin.

A growing number of women fill the posts of nursing-home administrator, medical director, physician, and other key positions that once were restricted to men. Similarly, a growing number of licensed nurses, nursing directors, and recreation leaders are men, where previously almost 100 percent of these positions were held by women. Here the administrator is referred to as male and the nursing director or nurse as female simply because the larger percentage of administrators are men and most nurses are women. This same basis of referral will be used in discussing all other nursing-home personnel. With the single exception that the *orderly* is the male counterpart of *aide*, every position in the nursing home is open to male or female personnel.

The administrator, through the department heads and their staffs, is ultimately responsible for everything that goes on within the nursing home: everything from the cleanliness of the patient's room, the tastiness of his meals, and his personal safety, all the way to such matters as ensuring the caliber of professional personnel in teaching an amputee to use prosthetic legs, educating a diabetic to the self-administration of intramuscular injections and the restrictions of his diet, and meeting the emotional, social, and spiritual needs of all patients, whether alert or disoriented.

The administrator's efforts toward formulating the best possible services and programs for the patients must be matched by his efforts to establish broad personnel policies and comprehensive orientation and training programs for employees. If he is wise, he realizes that only well-trained and contented employees can help him to achieve his goal of well-cared-for and contented patients.

He is responsible, too, for forms, procedures, manuals, reports, job descriptions, purchasing, fiscal management, and optimum community relations with other health-care facilities and social agencies, and with the residents of the nursing home's community.

As it is impractical to list here *all* the areas of administrative responsibility, only the highlights have been pinpointed. The administrator carries full responsibility for meeting all obligations, listed and unlisted. Working with him on one side are the owners or trustees, and on the other, the department heads and personnel.

Nursing-home administrators are state licensed (pages 15, 16). Many a nursing home, depending on its size and governmental regulations, has an assistant administrator who is also state licensed as an administrator.

Evaluating the administrator. It is only natural for you to be influenced by the administrator's personality: his warmth and friendly attitude, and his evident concern with you and with your patient. That is, of course, if you get to meet him. In many nursing homes you will never have this opportunity. However, if you do, don't be swayed by his manner. Of course he's interested. Your patient is a prospective customer and, in order to operate in the black, he must keep beds constantly occupied. Judge the administrator, rather, by the effective performance and the concerned attitudes of all the departments and all the employees of the home.

Few people are aware that they have the right to read government inspection reports on any licensed nursing home. These are available at the local social security, department of health, or department of welfare offices. You will be able to examine the details of every aspect of the nursing home that is governed by federal, state, and local regulations. Unless the facility is brand-new, read reports covering several years so that you can observe patterns: the types of deficiencies that are noted and how frequently they may occur. However, as much as you will learn of the safety and sanitation of the building, the qualifications and the numbers of personnel, and the range and the efficacy of services, these accounts will not refer to attitudes toward patients: whether they are treated with respect and concern or with total indifference.

Following are ten specific means of judging administrative practice of respect and regard for patients. These are listed at random, since order of importance is a matter of individual estimation.

1. *A patients' council clearly illustrates the level of administrative concern.* This group is comprised of patients who volunteer to serve as representatives of all the patients, and who meet at regular intervals, usually monthly or semimonthly. Council members elect their own chairman (and any other officers) and discuss their feelings about the nursing home and its programs and personnel and their ideas for change or improvement.

The council report is submitted directly to the administrator who is at least morally obligated to give it his full consideration and then discuss his response with the council or with the council's chairman. Surely council members lack the professional training and the necessary multifaceted perspective to establish policies. However, their experience as patients and as thinking persons can influence philosophies of the home and allow them to make such simple decisions as painting dayrooms yellow or blue or showing the weekly movie at a different hour so that it will not conflict with physical therapy sessions.

One administrator who instituted this type of council in his nursing home was immediately questioned by the owner as to whether or not the council was mandated for licensure. When he answered that it was not, the owner asked, "Then why are you sticking out your neck?" A concerned administrator does not consider it "sticking out his neck" to learn the patients' problems and suggestions. He recognizes that the home is being run for the benefit of the patients, and that an essential element in its success is meeting the desires and emotional needs of the patients as far as is humanly and professionally possible. The patients' council will bring those needs and wishes directly to him. He can work toward his objective of meeting the total needs of the patients only when he is fully aware of those needs.

When the patient population of a nursing home includes a significant number of young patients, as well as aged ones, then there should be two separate councils, each reflecting the thinking of its own peer group.

2. *Is there an established bedtime for all patients?* The simplest way to find a truthful answer to this is by asking some of the patients. Must everyone be in bed by nine o'clock, for instance, or six o'clock or sometimes even four in the afternoon? This is typical of the average nursing home but totally unnecessary. Its only advantage is for the nursing staff who are eager to complete their chores. Unless the patient's physician has prescribed a specific bedtime, why can't he read, write letters, converse socially, or watch the late show or even the late late show on television? The nursing home is indeed his home and will be for a period of months or years. Many nurses will understand, appreciate, and cooperate with this point of view. Many others will resent it, because it is certainly easier to have all the patients tucked away in bed at an early hour. You will know that you have met a patient-oriented administrator if he has issued the directive that, barring medical prescription to the contrary, patients are to be respected as adults in electing their own bedtimes.

It is, of course, an obvious truth that the earlier a patient goes to sleep at night, the earlier he is apt to awaken in the morning, and consequently, the sooner baths or showers will be completed and all the beds made. But what if some beds are not made until eleven o'clock or noon or one? And why can't patients be given the choice of bathing at night rather than in the morning? This can more nearly approximate normal routine for a number of patients and at the same time ease the workload for day-shift nursing personnel.

3. *Accent on safety is another manifestation of administrative concern.* Although it's a simple matter for you to find out if a safety committee exists, it will be considerably more difficult—perhaps impossible—for you to determine whether or not such a committee is active and interested, and how often it meets. But you will be able to observe for yourself the safety measures provided in the case of fire (page 28). Make it a point to notice whether or not all the beds have bedrails (they should), look for cracked window-panes, splinters in corridor handrails, torn carpet or tiling, burned out light bulbs, wheelchairs or other equipment in disrepair, chipped edges on glasses or dinnerware, doors that may open and close with difficulty, and other similar telltale signs. Determine if warning notices are placed at floor areas that are either freshly washed or freshly waxed.

4. *The administrator's availability to you and to your patient is a further indication of his attitude.* You cannot expect him to be available at any time that happens to be convenient to you, nor can you expect frequent interviews with him. Confine these interviews to matters of utmost importance and only after you have exhausted routine channels. You have read a brief review of his duties and must be aware that his time is heavily occupied. Despite this, a patient-oriented administrator will make time, whenever he can, to see patients on a one-to-one basis and

to see their relatives when they have pressing problems to discuss. Direct conversations centered around these problems will assist him to meet his goals of optimum total care for the total patient.

Established visiting hours should have flexibility to accommodate those persons who otherwise would be unable to visit.

5. *Liberal daily visiting hours, covering both afternoons and evenings, show recognition of the patients' social and emotional needs.* It's possible, but unlikely, to find the nursing home that offers unlimited visiting hours. This, of course, allows a husband or adult child to visit on his way to work in the morning or a young woman to plan her visits around the needs of her family at home. However, the average nursing facility will want mornings and mealtimes "undisturbed" by visitors, since these are the hours when staff members are busiest. Doors should always be open to children and infants as well as to adult relatives and friends. Contrary to the hospital that establishes a minimum age for visitors, generally 12 or 14, the nursing home is not concerned with acute illness and therefore need not prohibit youngsters from visiting. There is no justifiable reason for depriving the nursing-home patient of the inherent joy and comfort of frequent visits with beloved grandchildren or other children whom he may love.

6. *Some nursing homes allow cocktails or other alcoholic beverages to patients whose attending physicians write such prescriptions.* The average nursing-home patient has had to abandon most of his established life patterns. Why not preserve those that can be safely maintained?

One elderly gentleman admitted to a nursing home after major surgery showed no signs of progress. The center of the problem appeared to be his loss of appetite. Although he was repeatedly offered substitute foods, nothing tempted him. Finally he confessed that he missed the beer he had been accustomed to having with lunch and supper. His attending physician was contacted and wrote out a prescription permitting him up to two glasses of beer with each of these meals. The patient responded with a hearty appetite and a subsequent and steady improvement in his overall health status.

7. *A concerned and people-oriented administrator is eager to keep patients and relatives well informed.* To achieve this, one or all of the following can be put into effect:

Both patient and family members should be given a full orientation to the nursing home: a tour of the facility, a summary of services and staff members, and at least a brief presentation of objectives and attitudes. Beware of the nursing home that restricts your tour to one nursing area. This *could* be the only area fit to view.

Regularly scheduled family meetings, once a month—or even every two or three months—can be a productive administrative tool. Patients' relatives or close friends are invited to attend and to present questions or problems to the administrator or to department heads. *When these expressed opinions and viewpoints are heeded,* or when the family meeting is used to allow the staff—or consultants—the opportunity to indoctrinate the participants to nursing-home goals, to problems common to the aging or the handicapped, or to new developments in health legislation, these meetings can provide a significant learning experience to relatives and staff alike.

A mimeographed newsletter for patients, relatives, staff, and volunteers can be issued monthly or two or three times a year. It is a means of announcing new programs, new staff, and new or newly proposed health legislation, as well as events that take place within the home or special occasions in the lives of its patients or employees.

A small brochure tersely stating do's and don't's, when's and where's, and *patients' rights* should be distributed to all patients and their relatives or close friends.

All of the above points need careful scrutiny to determine whether they are merely public relations gimmicks or whether they represent honest administrative endeavor to teach, to learn, and consequently to improve the level of long-term care.

8. *Does the administrator give patients the opportunity to do?* The nursing-home patient is actually at the mercy of staff members who do for him and to him what he used to do for himself. Senator Pat McNamara once said in a report to the Senate on the Problems of the Aged and Aging that "Americans work not only to earn what is necessary to exist but to achieve a sense of purpose, to feel a belonging, to enjoy the pride of playing a role in the drama of life." This sense of purpose, belonging, and pride becomes more urgent with institutionalization. Patients can be given the opportunity and the *choice* of serving as volunteers in assuming such responsibilities as assorting or delivering patient mail, routine typing that does not divulge patient information or other confidential matters, carrying messages, counting silverware and setting tables, reading to more handicapped patients or feeding them, working in the library, arranging fresh flowers and changing their water for patients unable to perform for themselves, and working outdoors in the garden during the warm weather.

9. *Tipping must be a taboo in any nursing home.* To be fair, the administrator does not have direct control in preventing staff members from requesting tips or accepting them. However, he is to be heartily congratulated, as are his employees, if tips are refused and never solicited.

There are nursing homes where patients must tip to be toileted, to be bathed, to be fed. I know of one patient, a paraplegic, who told me with considerable pride that she had learned to control herself so that she needed toileting only twice a day. "Now I can get by for just fifty cents a day!" she exulted. Consider for a moment the indignity of always needing help to perform a natural function that would normally require no assistance whatever; now compound this affront to your ego by the humiliation of a hand outstretched for payment.

10. *Finally, there is an aura of warmth and contentment, or of stress and resentment, that pervades a nursing facility just as it does a personal residence.* Accuracy in judging this, or *feeling* it, depends largely on how reliable or how keenly developed your sensitivity is to an emotional undercurrent that is more revealing than words. Patients who are unhappy and intimidated are apt to fear reprisal by staff members on whom they depend, and so they say nothing at all or tell the easy lie that everything's just fine. A strong intuition, or the ability to communicate without the use of words, may help you to discern the prevalent attitudes of patients and personnel.

The Medical Director

From the time of its inception, the licensed skilled nursing facility had not been required by federal law to hire a medical director but had been permitted to function with the services of an advisory physician who carried some of the responsibilities of the medical director, but not all, and gave considerably less time to the facility. However, many well-run homes of appreciable size have had part-time medical directors on staff, and many states have required a medical director as a qualification for state licensure.

At long last the post of medical director has become a requirement for federal licensure. (Consideration is given to the more rural areas where continued effort fails to fill this post. In this event the skilled nursing facility is permitted to operate with the services of an advisory physician, as it has done in the past.)

A state-licensed physician of medicine or osteopathy must serve as medical director on either a part-time or full-time basis. This regulation became effective on December 2, 1974, although the final target date for filling the requirement was set for a full year later. An organized medical staff, with approval of the governing body, may elect the facility's medical director, or medical direction can be provided to a group of facilities through a local medical society, hospital medical staff, or other medical group. A hospital-based nursing facility may have a member of that hospital's medical staff serve as medical director.

Although a medical director on staff will not assure you of optimum patient care, it is likely that he will provide for medical and medically related services that are more professional in quality. One of the great hazards to be overcome in the medical care of nursing-home patients is the inclination on the part of many physicians to be disinterested in elderly and chronically ill patients. They tend to regard them as uninteresting and unchallenging, with the theory that they'll never achieve full recovery anyhow. The personal attitude and the professional caliber of the medical director are all-important in influencing the many areas that come under his immediate and general jurisdiction. It would be wise for you to determine what you can about his reputation, his background, his relationships with patients, and his hospital affiliations.

The time that the medical director devotes to this position is separate and apart from whatever hours he may give to his personal patients residing in the facility and is reimbursed by the home on a salary basis. In addition to establishing and enforcing medical policies, he develops written by-laws and rules and regulations, including the delineation of attending physicians' responsibilities, which must be approved by the governing body. He supervises and coordinates all medical and medically related programs, such as rehabilitation services, pharmacy, laboratory, and X ray, and works closely with the nursing and dietary departments. His responsibilities include the recruitment and general supervision of a staff of well-qualified attending physicians, as well as a dentist, podiatrist, and optometrist for regular routine services, and consultants in all the major specialties. Although the services of consultants, podiatrist, and optometrist are not federal requirements, they are compulsory under a number of state codes and are essential to the comprehensive and thorough medical management of the patient.

In addition to assuming responsibility for medical administration, the medical director works with the home's administrator in determining employee health policies and in supervising the occupational health status of staff members and the environmental health factors of the physical plant. He reviews all accidents occurring to patients, employees, or visitors on the premises of the nursing home in order to pinpoint areas that may be hazardous to health and safety. Such incidents are immediately referred to the charge nurse, and a written report is promptly completed in detail and signed by any witnesses and by the examining physician or licensed nurse. When the accident occurs to a patient, the report is maintained as a permanent part of his medical record and copies are sent to the administrator and to the state licensing agency. All reports of accidents—whether to patients, employees, or visitors—are studied by the medical director, the safety committee, and, frequently, by the in-service education director in an effort to reduce their causes. Duplicates of the reports are filed together as a unit and maintained for inspection by regulatory agencies.

The medical director is obligated to provide for full-time emergency coverage by attending physicians and/or himself. To this end a written schedule of physicians to be called in case of emergency is made readily available to the nursing staff, as are written policies for control of communicable diseases.

The Attending Physician

The attending physician is your patient's personal doctor. He may or may not be the medical director as well, but this will have no effect on his role as attending physician.

The patient, or patient's relative, should be given free choice of attending physician as a personal right, although this is not a legal requirement. Frequently the nursing facility confines the patient's choice to its staff physicians; if a patient chooses another physician, however, it is likely that the home will allow that doctor to apply for staff membership. The right to change doctors at any time and for any reason should also be viewed as a personal right, and generally is. The patient or his responsible relative must assume full responsibility for effecting such a change: for discontinuing the services of one physician and taking on the services of another. These two actions need to be well coordinated, since the patient must be under the care of a physician *at all times.* If the physician chosen for replacement is not a member of the nursing home's medical staff, then it becomes essential to discuss the plan with the administrator before any steps are taken. If the physician is a member of the staff, the head nurse or nursing supervisor must be notified promptly. She, in turn, will alert administrative personnel.

The attending physician has the obligation of keeping his patient apprised of medical treatment, progress, and any change in his health status. If the patient is not mentally alert, then this right falls to his closest relative or friend. The attending physician has the legal obligation of planning (and entering in the patient's medical chart) both short- and long-term health and rehabilitation goals and monthly reviews of medications, treatments, and general progress.

The medical charts are accurately maintained, classified as confidential, and preserved by the facility for a minimum period of five years (or longer in some states). In the case of minors they must be preserved until the patient is at least 24 years old.

The attending physician has the further responsibility of formulating specific written discharge plans. These are initiated within the first seven days of the patient's admission to the facility and are updated at regular intervals by the physician and other professionals directly concerned with the patient's care.

The doctor has unique problems in caring for a nursing-home patient. For your own peace of mind, and your patient's, it is important to understand these special problems.

According to federal regulations, an attending physician must visit his nursing-home patient once a month, but, barring an emergency, his visits are limited to once a month only. Government agencies are allowed wide and arbitrary interpretation of what constitutes an emergency. Frequently they disagree with the physician's determination and thus disallow reimbursement.

Occasionally, following the first ninety days after admission, the attending physician may request and be granted authorization to visit the patient as little as every sixty days. This change can be effected only when he justifies and documents that the patient's physical condition no longer warrants monthly visits, and only in the event that the patient does not require regularly administered rehabilitation treatment. In the case of a Medicare or Medicaid patient, the alternate schedule of physician visits at sixty-day intervals must be approved by the utilization review committee (Chapter 8) whose members then reevaluate the patient's need for continued stay in the skilled nursing facility. Also, the appropriate agency (for Medicare or Medicaid) must be notified immediately, and again the patient's need for skilled nursing care is reevaluated, this time by the agency's medical team.

If your patient is covered by Medicare or Medicaid, or both, his attending physician will be constantly harassed by (1) governmental establishment of the fee he is permitted to charge, usually an amount less than his current fee for an office visit; (2) long and detailed forms for billing Medicare or Medicaid (in many instances, both), compounded by the recurrent need to remit duplicate billing, and often a wait of many months for reimbursement; and (3) the improbability of collecting payment for more than one visit monthly (or sometimes bimonthly).

Your response to all this may well be that doctors are doing all right for themselves; they make plenty of money, and you can hardly concern yourself with whether or not they are inconvenienced by Medicare or Medicaid requirements. Certainly, you say, they are not depending on *you* for maintaining their homes and families, running their cars, or paying for well-equipped offices and secretarial or nursing help. But they *are* depending on you, the collective you, not only for the expenses mentioned but for the escalating costs of living, of payroll, and —particularly—the costs of medical liability insurance that are increasing at an incredible rate.

In America we are heading toward some form of national health insurance geared to guarantee comprehensive medical care to every citizen. Such a program might well be administered and even partially funded by individual states, but all signs point toward federalized standards. Both preventive medicine and health maintenance are the inherent rights of human beings, and this is gradually being recognized by the federal government. Medicare and Medicaid provide some of the answers to the problems but far from all.

Here is an example of what these two existing programs mean to physicians today. Three doctors practice together in an upstate county of New York. Two of them are internists; the third is a general practitioner. They have shared their practice for more than ten years, and together they care for over half the population of that county. Initially they employed two women. One was a full-time receptionist and nurse; the second came in one and a half days a week to do billing and bookkeeping. Today, because of the vast amount of paper work and duplication required by Medicare and Medicaid, these same three physicians employ seven women full-time. Thus the cost of running their office has risen sharply. Their income, however, has dropped because of the smaller fees approved for Medicare and Medicaid patients, the growing number of patients enjoying these benefits, and also because it is next to impossible to collect any monies from either of these programs for more than one monthly visit to the steadily increasing number of patients confined to nursing homes.

Another example: A doctor made his routine monthly visit to a nursing-home patient. Exactly three days later she suddenly developed a fever of 104.2. The nurse telephoned the physician to report the temperature, and he responded in the only way he could. He came directly to the nursing home to see his patient.

At this writing eleven months have passed. The patient referred to is covered by Medicare Parts A and B and by Medicaid. The doctor has not been reimbursed by Medicare since it was their decision that this visit was not necessary. After all, the doctor had seen her just three days earlier. According to governmental procedure, he cannot bill Medicaid until or unless the examination of that patient is first approved and then proportionately reimbursed by Medicare.

In this particular case, the doctor has decided to invest whatever time and effort is required to continue to follow up the matter. He has no doubt that his second visit was essential. Should he finally collect his fee, which at this time seems extremely unlikely, it will have cost him considerably more by way of secretarial time and pure aggravation than his fee is worth, but he has determined to break through the obstacle of the arbitrary allowance of one visit a month.

If your patient has been admitted to the nursing home on a private basis (no Medicare or Medicaid) and all his bills are being paid directly by him or by a member of the family, certainly the question of the doctor's visits will be greatly simplified. But it won't do away with the problem altogether. Consider that a doctor's time and know-how are the source of his livelihood, that any doctor of merit and good standing is actively working about twelve hours out of every twenty-four. These hours are divided among regular daily visits to his acutely ill patients in the hospital, office hours, emergencies, studying medical journals and articles so that he can keep abreast of new developments, and, generally, involvement with special committees at his hospital and local medical society, and teaching.

It is for a combination of all these reasons that most physicians have been forced to curtail or completely eliminate house calls. The time involved in coming and going is time taken away from other patients and attendant obligations. The physician's monthly visit to the nursing home is an occasion when he can visit all of his patients who are confined there. When he comes to visit your patient on other than a monthly basis—when the visit is to your patient alone—then he is, in fact, making a house call.

Your probable reaction to all of this? Your primary concern is your patient. When he's sick you want medical attention for him, and you want it right then and there. So does everyone. It is for this very reason that the doctor's dilemma has been presented here. It is a fact of life that must be met by every nursing-home patient—private, Medicare, or Medicaid—and by everyone whose peace of mind is affected by that patient's well-being.

The attending physician or, in his absence, the medical director has the right to give your patient permission to leave the nursing home when he is accompanied by a qualified adult who will sign responsibility for him. This leave can be for a few hours, for a weekend at home, or longer. If your patient is private, he will have to pay for his bed while he is away. If he is covered by Medicare or Medicaid, specific rulings apply as to how many hours or days his bed can be held for him. Medicaid regulations vary in different states.

Evaluating the Medical Department. This is literally impossible unless you, too, are a physician. Assuming that you are not, the only yardsticks at your disposal are some of the areas of medical responsibility. Are the rehabilitation services well run and is equipment modern, well maintained, and varied? Are there consultants in the major specialties? Are dental, podiatric, and optometric services readily available whenever your patient may require them? Does the attending physician visit your patient at regularly established intervals? Is he or a substitute physician always on call for emergencies?

These are probably the only evaluation tools available to you, other than the reputation and affiliations of the physician who serves as medical director or advisory physician and of those who serve on the medical staff of the home as attending physicians and as consultants.

5

Yardsticks:
Nursing and Dietary

Nursing Services

THE BASIC GOAL of the nursing department is comprehensive, high quality professional care covering all aspects of restorative nursing and precision in following medical orders. Obligation is not limited to physical care, but extends to the emotional well-being of the patient, good grooming, assistance in the activities of daily living, and the coordination of nursing care with all other services and treatments. In order to fully achieve these objectives, all nursing personnel need to know their patients individually and recognize their varying needs.

The Nursing Director

The director of nursing has the responsibility for meeting these requirements. She is responsible for adhering to all federal, state, and local regulations that pertain to nursing and for the effective performance of every member of her staff. She reports directly to the administrator and is free to consult with the medical director for guidance, direction, and medical information. The nursing director frequently has an assistant, depending on the number of patients in the home and the requirements of the licensing agencies. In the temporary absence of the nursing director (and assistant), the nursing supervisor is in charge of the department. If there is no supervisor, then the obligation is met by the charge nurse.

Restorative Nursing

Many nursing-home patients are institutionalized for weeks or months of convalescence following illness or surgery. When recovery is achieved, they are discharged from the facility. Many other nursing-home patients never recover and continue to need professional care over a period of years, frequently the remainder of their lifetimes. A primary goal of the nursing home—and of all employees concerned with patient care—is to restore to every patient the highest level of physical and emotional independence of which he is individually capable. This can be complete independence and discharge to home. It can be a moderate level of independence and transfer to an intermediate care facility. It may be that independence cannot be achieved at all and that the only realistic goal is maintenance of minimal function. Restorative services (including medicine, nursing, rehabilitation therapies, dietary, recreation, and social service) work together toward the common objective of helping the patient to help himself.

Restorative nursing (sometimes referred to as rehabilitative nursing) is a comprehensive and requisite function of the nursing department. It includes simple basic tasks, such as frequently turning paralyzed or otherwise bedridden patients to help avoid bedsores, and supplementing physical, occupational, and speech therapies in regular practical help with the activities of daily living: combing hair, brushing teeth, eating, ambulating, simple conversation, and similar activities that most of us take for granted.

The key to restorative nursing is motivation. The patient

must be motivated to help himself or significant rehabilitation cannot be realized. He must want to do for himself, to develop an interest in his appearance and in social activities, and to join in the cooperative effort to restore some or all of the functions he has lost. Socialization is an important tool in patient motivation. Nurses and aides have more contact with patients than any other staff members of the home. Thus it behooves them to try to interest and encourage patients to participate in recreation programs, to join others in the dayroom or dining room, and to keep themselves clean and well groomed.

One aspect of staff attitude toward patients concerns sex. The popular belief that sex has no place in institutional living or in the lives of the aged, disabled, or infirm could not be further from the truth. The sex urge persists except in some rare cases of excessive physical or mental debilitation. Denial of fulfillment is but one more on the long list of frustrations suffered by institutionalized patients.

Obviously there cannot be freedom of sex in any institution. But there are exceptions to every rule. I was serving in my capacity as nursing-home administrator when a charge nurse came to me and said in shocked tones, "Do you know that Mr. Hughes was in Miss Winters' bedroom last night? And I hear that it happens all the time. What should we *do?*" I'm sure that she expected me to join in her indignation. I didn't. Mr. Hughes was a 52-year-old bachelor, crippled through an illness during his adolescence, and living now in a four-bedded room of the home. Miss Winters, a spinster in her late 50s, was suffering the early stages of premature senility. She enjoyed the privacy of a single-bedded room. Had she shared a room with another patient, my response would have differed in deference to her roommate. Under these circumstances, however, I told the confused and red-faced charge nurse that the thing to do was to keep the door closed and to be sure not to let anyone enter the room unless Mr. Hughes or Miss Winters called for help.

Two people were enjoying a little time of natural living,

hurting nobody, and offending only those who, like the reporting charge nurse, might take it upon themselves to act as judge
and jury.

Many patients relegated to institutional living find that the
easiest path is return to the womb: inertia, submission, and
total acceptance. Many nurses and other staff members accept
this passivity. They prefer a parent-child relationship with
the patient and feel threatened when he approaches independence. They either fail to understand or choose to ignore that
care and concern can be administered on a level of equality as
with husband and wife. It is anything but easy to remotivate a
resigned, phlegmatic patient. It requires time, devotion, and
resolution. In some cases it can never be achieved, but in the
many instances of success, rewards are infinite for the patient
and for the personnel who work together to achieve it.

Family members and friends play an invaluable role in re-
motivating patients. It's so easy for a patient to give up if he
feels that nobody cares. There's a reason to work and to try if
he can anticipate the reward of pleasing a loved one or if he
can look forward to discharge from the nursing home and re-
joining his family and society. Many patients are neglected or
even abandoned by family and friends and thus pose an infinitely greater problem or challenge (depending on the point of
view) to the nursing staff. When aides or nurses find some spare
moments, playing cards or checkers with a patient or just chat-
ting can be as fundamental to his needs as bathing him or
bringing him fresh drinking water. It is within the wide scope
of restorative nursing to make it a practice to call a patient by
name (hopefully his last name unless he has specifically requested otherwise), to talk with him about any matters that
arouse his interest; to give him personal recognition by remem-
bering his likes and dislikes, by asking about what happened in
physical therapy that morning or if he enjoyed the movie he
watched on television last night.

Of the two incidents that follow, one illustrates a positive approach to remotivation and restorative nursing, and the other negates it completely.

The first example concerns a patient and an aide, a Mrs. Phillips and a Miss Adams. Mrs. Phillips was a widow in her mid-70s who was confined to a nursing home because of severe Parkinson's disease. She had no family and no visitors.

She was seriously incapacitated by her illness and excessively self-conscious of its manifestations. Her head was unsteady on her neck, and her arms shook violently when she made an effort to use them. When she walked—which she could do only with assistance—her gait was unsteady and she appeared to be pitching forward, as though she would fall at any minute. Her voice had been reduced to a mere whisper, and conversation with her required intense concentration. She was a private patient in a private room. She remained in that room all day, every day, sometimes in bed and sometimes sitting up in her armchair. The nursing staff attempted to coax her to the day-room to socialize with other patients or to attend recreation programs or go to the dining room for her meals. She refused. She sat all day alone, unoccupied and totally unmotivated.

Miss Adams, a young aide, took an interest in Mrs. Phillips. Whenever she had five or ten minutes between chores, she went into Mrs. Phillips' room. During her first several visits she found that Mrs. Phillips ignored any conversation, so Miss Adams simply sat in the room with her, picked up a magazine to look at and, after a few minutes, left and went about her business. Then one day she asked if she might turn on the little bedside radio. Mrs. Phillips nodded her head in approval. Soon the two sat together listening to music or news programs. Occasionally Mrs. Phillips would glance at the magazine that Miss Adams held in her hands. After several more weeks Miss Adams began to read aloud, and Mrs. Phillips appeared interested. It took months of this simple acceptance on the part of a new friend until one morning Mrs. Phillips agreed to go out into the corridor with Miss Adams. Once she left her room, it was only a matter of days until she had the confidence to go to the dining room, the dayroom, and the movies.

This is indicative of the kind of remotivation essential to putting patients on the road toward an incentive for living and recovery of function. This is restorative nursing at its best. It provides the ingredient of personal concern necessary to encourage the patient to self-help.

The second and negative example concerns a 20-year-old man who, at his own request, was always addressed by his first name, Tom. Tom was a victim of multiple sclerosis. His arms and legs had become so stiffened as to be utterly useless to him. His speech was so poor that the only way to understand him was to ask him to spell out what it was that he wanted. Slowly and painstakingly he would mouth the letters W . . . A . . . T . . . , and suddenly you realized he was asking for water. He was pleasant and sweet and outgoing. Aides and orderlies and volunteers propelled him in his wheelchair to the dining room, to passive recreation programs, to the porch or library or lobby.

During my early years of working as a department head, I was making rounds one evening with the nursing supervisor, a Mrs. Lester. As we approached Tom's bed, Mrs. Lester told me that they had started to stretch Tom's legs every day in an attempt to keep them from becoming stiffer than they already were. She explained that this was a medically prescribed treatment, essential but painful. When we arrived at Tom's bedside, he looked up at Mrs. Lester and opened his mouth to speak. Mrs. Lester anticipated his words, looked down at him, and stated firmly and briskly, "We're going to stretch your legs tomorrow and the next day and the day after that, so get used to it," and then she abruptly walked away. I looked at Tom. Mrs. Lester had gone. Time had been too short for him to ask her anything, tell her anything. His eyes were filled with fright and bewilderment. The moment was over, and he was left alone with his questions and forebodings and anxieties.

Remotivation? Hardly. The message had come across loud

and clear: "We're interested in your legs, but we are not interested in you."

Volunteers. Volunteers supplement restorative nursing
through the unique role they play in motivating patients. They
represent the community outside the nursing home. They
prove their concern for the patient by the simple act of being
there. And they have the time to devote to individual patients
that daily job pressures deny to staff members.

Patient-Care Plans. Individual patient-care plans (formerly
called nursing-care plans) constitute an effective tool toward
patient-centered care. These written plans are maintained by
members of the nursing staff as well as all other disciplines familiar with the needs and the care of the individual patient.
The plans specify long- and short-term goals for every pertinent
area of the patient's professional care, and include his emotional, social, and rehabilitative needs as well as physical. They
serve as an excellent means of communication between nursing
shifts, present a simple tool for patient-care evaluation and discharge planning, and should help to insure personalized care,
provided they are updated at monthly or, preferably, weekly
intervals.

Patient Education. A further function of the nursing department, frequently pinpointed by the patient-care plan, is
the education of patients to a full understanding of their
health needs, especially in preparing them to return home or
for transfer to an intermediate care facility. Such teaching may
relate to the care of colostomies, optimum usage of false limbs,
general independence in the activities of daily living, or other
matters requiring instruction.

Medical Records. The patient-care plan is not to be confused with his medical record. The medical record or medical
chart is comprised of written long- and short-term goals and re-

ports of treatments, prescriptions, and progress in all the areas of professional care that concern him: medical, nursing, dietary, rehabilitation, social service, recreation, medical consultation, dentistry, podiatry, optometry, X ray, laboratory, and just about everything that has bearing on his physical, social, and emotional status. It presents a complete sociomedical patient profile that serves to mutually assist all professionals associated with patient care, implement discharge planning, and provide full information should the time arrive for patient transfer.

Medications. One of the chief responsibilities of the nursing department is the administration of medications in accordance with physicians' orders. It frequently occurs that patients or their relatives are plagued with questions concerning these medications and with the denial of requests for "something, please" to relieve a headache or nausea or sleeplessness.

Let me attempt to answer the more common of these problems.

When your patient has been taking X-Y-Z pills for the past three years and must continue to take them, why can't you bring in the half-full bottle from his medicine chest? Why must you buy a new prescription? And later, if Mrs. Evans down the corridor has been on the same medication but now no longer needs it, why can't your patient have her unused pills instead of purchasing another bottle?

The answers to these questions are imposed by law and not by the administrator or the medical or nursing director. When a patient is admitted directly from a hospital some states allow him to bring medications that were provided to him by the hospital during the course of his stay. However, he may never bring medications from home. The nursing home shoulders full responsibility for his care, and the only way that it can ascertain "beyond the shadow of a doubt" that no substitution has been made is to either give his prescription directly to a pharmacy or have evidence that this has been done by the hospital. When the patient is discharged from the nursing home, he may take his medications with him only if the attending physician or medical director enters specific written permission on his medical chart.

The answer to why the patient can't use Mrs. Evans' prescription, which was filled by the nursing home's pharmacy, is likewise a matter of legal restriction but considerably more difficult to understand. The law states that any medication unused by the patient for whom it was initially prescribed must be destroyed and the destruction recorded. Why, I don't know. I've never met anyone who does know.

Every nursing home works with the services of a consultant pharmacist. Occasionally a nursing home enjoys the advantages of a pharmacy on the premises manned by a staff pharmacist. In such an instance the patient reaps substantial benefit. His attending physician need not order fifty or one hundred tablets of any medication. The pharmacist maintains a full stock of drugs and sends the prescribed quantity of tablets, liquids, or injectables to the nursing station each day. If the physician sees fit to change medication for the patient, there is no surplus to be destroyed, and no cost to the patient for unused medicine. Such an arrangement, however, is the exception and not the rule. Usually all drugs, narcotics and others, are ordered from a local pharmacy and are kept under lock and key at the nursing station. Incidentally, the patient has the legal right to choice of pharmacy.

Although you and your patient may be accustomed to taking an aspirin or vitamin tablet whenever you please, a nurse may give no medication, however mild, without the specific prescription of the attending physician, consultant, or medical director. She is not being unconcerned or ruthless when she denies your patient those aspirins. She jeopardizes her license and your patient's health unless she has the physician's specific prescription. In an emergency she can telephone your patient's doctor. She must then enter the prescription on your patient's medical chart, and this prescription must be countersigned within forty-eight hours by either the issuing physician or the medical director.

Except for doctors, only licensed nurses (and occasionally other staff members who have satisfactorily completed special state-approved courses) are permitted to administer medications. The medication nurse is required to watch the patient swallow his medications (so that he cannot store them or discard them) and enter the information on his personal medication card. Any error in medication must be reported immediately to the patient's physician and the nursing director, and a full report must be written and maintained in the patient's medical record

Narcotics are counted at each change of shift so that the charge nurse coming on duty at four o'clock in the afternoon, for instance, has an exact count from the nurse she is relieving. A permanent record is kept of these computations. Unused narcotics, after accurate count, are returned to the regional department of health or other authorized state agency and, as a double check, are destroyed on those premises.

Staffing the Nursing Department. Federal regulations call for a registered nurse to serve as nursing director on a full-time basis, a registered staff nurse on day duty seven days a week, and either registered or practical nurses to serve as charge nurses around-the-clock. In some sparsely populated areas where a minimum number of registered nurses are available, a facility is permitted to have one staff nurse only, covering five days a week rather than seven. Other than this, regulations demand "a sufficient number of qualified nursing personnel to meet the total nursing needs of all patients." This includes nurses, aides, orderlies, and ward clerks.

The determination of the number of licensed nurses considered to be "sufficient," the determination of criteria for "qualified" nursing personnel, and the determination of "the total nursing needs of all patients" are sometimes stipulated by state requirements. However, when state regulations are lower than federal, or equal to them, then these determinations are left to the discretion of the licensing agency. A number of states are specific in their demands for qualifications of nursing personnel, the ratio of their numbers to the needs of the patients, and the ratio of licensed to unlicensed personnel. But even then, staffing is based on average patient needs throughout the state and does not take into account the individual nursing home whose unique patient population may require more hours of nursing care than the average figures allow.

All of this may or may not have serious consequences for your patient. If he is one of the more fortunate, if his needs require limited nursing time, there is no problem. If, however, your patient is paralyzed or is suffering from a chronic disease such as multiple sclerosis or muscular dystrophy or is in the terminal stages of spinal cancer, he will then require considerable nursing care each day. Your probable reaction is that his needs will average out with those of patients who require substantially less care. The fact is, however, that the nursing home will be loath to admit him at all. The average nursing home looks for those patients with minimum care requirements because of the problems of staffing. Approximately 90 percent of all nursing-home patients are covered by Medicare, Medicaid, or both, and reimbursement schedules are established by government agencies on an approved cost-plus basis. Results show that many nursing-home beds are given to patients with minimum time-consuming problems (both physical and emotional) and are denied to those patients who have the greater need for nursing care and the attendant therapeutic services of the nursing home.

A paradoxical problem arises with the stated purpose of the utilization review committee discussed in Chapter 8.

In-Service Education. Federal requirements call for an inservice education director (who need not be a nurse) to shoulder the responsibility for planning, scheduling, and manning an on-going training and education program for all members of staff. This includes orientation to the nursing home and its policies and training geared to the needs of the aged, ill, and disabled. It covers infection prevention and control, safety, confidentiality of patient information, and respect for the patient's dignity, privacy, and personal belongings.

A more valuable and comprehensive program, mandated by a number of states, calls for a registered nurse to serve as in-service director either on a full-time or part-time basis. Frequently the program is implemented by groups of homes combining their resources.

In addition to covering the material outlined above, the in-service director provides training to licensed nurses in current nursing approaches to the physical and psychological care of patients and keeps them informed of pertinent new developments in medicine, rehabilitation, and dietetics. She conducts many of these sessions herself, but also calls on physicians in the various specialties, therapists, key medical and nursing consultants in the community, and department heads within the nursing home.

I would like to see greater emphasis on psychiatric training; and an active program of exchanging nurses (on a visiting basis only) with local general hospitals, specialty hospitals, rehabilitation centers, houses for the aged, etc., in order to broaden the perspective and the understanding of all nurses.

The in-service director gives aides and orderlies training in such procedures as bed-making, taking and recording blood pressures, temperatures, pulse and respiration rates; effective assistance in feeding and ambulating handicapped patients; routine turning in bed of paralyzed or semi-paralyzed patients; grooming of patients; escort service; understanding and contributing to nursing reports; and when to call for the assistance of a licensed nurse.

The quality of this education program is fundamental to the structure and the operation of a competent and concerned nursing department. The degree of its effectiveness is directly manifested by the degree of proficiency in the nursing care of your patient.

Evaluating the Nursing Department. By all means, judge the effectiveness of the nursing department by the quality of its care and the attitude of its personnel, but *don't* judge it by the number of its staff members. A licensed nursing home must meet the standards imposed by governmental agencies, and you will be guilty of wishful thinking if you expect it to provide more than that. Even if you feel that the number of nursing personnel is insufficient, plan on finding a still smaller number on weekends and holidays. This is as unavoidable in the nursing home as it is in the hospital. Many staff members wake up ill on a Sunday morning (either virus or baseball), and it is infinitely more difficult to find a replacement on short notice during weekends and holidays. All employees today enjoy liberal sick days, vacation, and holiday time. Face the fact that Susan Carter has a dozen valid reasons why she doesn't want to work on this particular Sunday or possibly Christmas morning. She has time coming to her, and she has decided to use it today. It may put your patient in an unhappy position, but it's Susan Carter's routine job, day in and day out, and on this particular morning she has placed her husband or her daughter or herself ahead of your patient. She's a great aide, or a great nurse, but she, too, is a human being with human frailties as well as strengths.

Judging the nursing department by the quality of its professional performance is a difficult task if you are not a physician or a nurse. But you can evaluate it to a large extent by the comfort and cleanliness of patients and by the staff's personal attitudes toward them. Be on the lookout for telltale signs. Spend time with several of the senile patients, the ones who cannot speak up for themselves to make demands. Notice their fingernails: Are they trim and clean? Is hair freshly shampooed? Are the men freshly shaven? Are incontinent patients soiled and wet or are they kept clean and dry? Are the patients in hospital garb wearing slippers on their feet? Are inordinate numbers of patients restrained to beds or wheelchairs? (Restraints may be used on medical prescription *only*.) Is there a bowel and bladder training program for incontinents?

Are the majority of patients wearing street clothing to help them retain self-identity? Are dresses and slacks and shirts clean and neat? Do some of the women have long, ugly hairs growing from their chins or have these been removed? Are eyeglasses clean? Are call-bells answered promptly? Is mealtime supervised by a licensed nurse? Are the patient's activities well coordinated, and does he understand what they are, and when, and why? Are patients' bed linens clean? (Linen won't be changed on a daily basis unless the patient is incontinent. Usually twice a week is the most you can expect.) Is there a covered pitcher of water and a clean glass always on the bedside table? Are the surfaces of these tables kept in orderly fashion?

A word of caution about the wheelchair patient who is slowly, slowly pushing her way toward the dayroom, and no nurse or aide comes to her assistance. Or the palsied patient who must summon his full concentration to feed himself while an aide is standing by idly, not offering help. *Don't* prejudge.

The second or third day that I ever worked in a nursing home, I was rushing along a corridor, fearing I would be late to my first department head meeting. On my way I passed an elderly woman seated in a wheelchair alongside a water cooler. She held a paper cup in a hand that shook relentlessly, and she was attempting to fill the cup. I stopped and asked, "May I help you?" Throughout the years I have clearly recalled her expression of unadulterated anger as she whipped out the single word "No!" I recognized then that the doing of something for oneself can have infinitely more meaning than the speed or adeptness of the doing. It can provide dignity and independence that are worth far more than help.

So don't jump to the conclusion that an employee is unconcerned if he doesn't offer assistance. Often it is better to wait to be asked; and, mostly, staff comes to know which patients welcome assistance and which ones prefer a measure of self-sufficiency.

It's a good idea to come back for a return visit when you are unexpected. If your initial visit to the nursing home was at ten in the morning, drop by at five or six in the evening. By all means, plan one of your visits at mealtime.

Dietary Department

The goal of the dietary department is to serve appetizing, healthful, and attractive meals, to adhere accurately to all dietary restrictions and needs prescribed for patients, and to educate patients to their own dietary requirements. Meals served in a nursing home, however, must do more than fill empty stomachs and follow dietary prescriptions. They must provide special times of day to be anticipated with pleasure.

Three meals a day should be served at reasonable times, with a lapse of no more than fourteen hours between supper and the next morning's breakfast. I fail to see where breakfast at 6 A.M. and supper at 4 P.M. provide any advantage over serving these same meals at 8 A.M. and 6 P.M. The only real difference is the measure of concern in helping to maintain or to further disrupt a patient's normal way of life. The early breakfast hour (which then, in turn, demands early lunch, early supper, and early-to-bed) is often explained as necessary so that the night staff can serve this meal, thus relieving the workload of the day staff, which carries the burden of most of the nursing duties. Breakfast at six in the morning, however, means being awakened at five; and the entire time readjustment can reach a point of absurdity.

An adequate interval should be allowed for the leisurely enjoyment of meals. In some nursing homes, trays are removed twenty minutes after they are delivered, thus forcing many patients to gulp their meals or to leave them unfinished.

Between-meal snacks should be served in midafternoon and again during the evening. A refrigerator belongs at each nursing station for the purpose of storing these snacks as well as patient-name-designated packages of food brought to the patients by their visitors. Incidentally, it is imperative that this refrigerator be used for foods only and in no way combined with the refrigerator used for storing medications.

The dietary department is run either by a full-time professional dietitian or by a chef-manager responsible to a part-time consultant dietitian. The dietitian is responsible directly to the administrator, works closely with nursing and medical departments, and has frequent and regular contact with all the patients.

A consultant dietitian is responsible for the planning of all menus, regular and special diets, and establishing dietary procedures. She participates in in-service education and training programs for the nursing department, develops and conducts in-service training programs for dietary personnel, and educates patients to their special dietary needs. An important part of her duties is the recording of patients' food likes and dislikes and arranging for substitutes when their dislikes are a part of the menu.

The chef-manager has a dual responsibility: to the consultant dietitian and to the administrator. It is he who shoulders the responsibility for meeting the sanitary standards of local and state health departments and for storing foods at proper temperatures and away from nonedible supplies. He schedules and supervises personnel within the department and is accountable for preparing all meals and snacks and insuring that they are delivered to patient floors and dining rooms at proper temperatures and under strictly sanitary conditions.

Descriptions of both these jobs are purposely sketchy in the belief that you are interested in only those duties that directly affect your patient.

When the dietitian serves on a full-time basis rather than in a consultant capacity only, she carries total responsibility for everything that goes on in the department and takes over the function of manager as well.

Evaluating the Dietary Department. I'd like to be able to tell you to judge the dietary department by your patient's response to his meals. Obviously that's not practical, because even the finest restaurants in the country cannot satisfy all their customers. Besides, the nursing home has a food budget to meet, and also your patient may be on a special diet. Judge the dietary services, rather, by whether or not the food is served under sanitary conditions and at proper temperatures; by whether the patient who is forbidden spices is served his spaghetti with no sauce at all (meaning "who cares?") or if he is given a substitute sauce or a substitute meal. Are his food likes and dislikes observed and are snacks pleasant and tasty? Are substitutes always available for him? Are holidays observed by special dinners and decorative place mats or small favors? Ask to see a cycle of menus. They may not particularly appeal to you, because they *can't* appeal to everybody, but determine if they're at all imaginative: try to picture the colors represented by meat, vegetable, and starch; take note of diversity in menus. Find out if there are different sets of menus for the winter and summer months. There should be.

Don't look for the impossible. It's a waste of your time and everyone else's. You will definitely not find Utopia, but hopefully you will find a nursing home where TLC (tender loving care) is a fact and not a fantasy.

6

Yardsticks:
Recreation, Rehabilitation,
and Social Services

Recreation

RECREATION HAS a twofold goal: as an end unto itself and as a means toward helping the patient achieve a sense of self-worth. It allows him to accomplish, to socialize, and to look forward to tomorrow. It allows him to exercise his God-given rights to *choose* and to *do*. The program does not require medical prescription, so the patient has the choice of whether or not he cares to participate at all, and he has the further choice of which activity he elects to join. Out of the endless hours of being done for and done to, he has the opportunity to do for himself.

Many years ago I decided to crochet an afghan, although I had never held a crochet needle in my hand. A friend offered her help, but I had a better idea. One day when I had a few spare minutes I brought some wool and a crochet needle to a paraplegic patient who was skilled in handiwork, and asked her if she would be good enough to teach me to crochet. Of course she said yes, as I knew she would or I wouldn't have asked. I drew up a chair next to her wheelchair, and she started by showing me how to hold the needle, how to hold the wool, how to make a simple chain stitch. Only a few minutes had passed when a nurse came into the room. The patient lifted her head and shouted to the nurse, "Look, *she's* taking, *I'm* giving!"

Schedules of active and passive programs are designed to meet the varying interests and potentials of the patients: activities such as wheelchair bowling, miniature golf, shuffle-board, dart-throwing (rubber tipped darts and a bull's-eye poster), games with a beach ball or a beanbag, sing-alongs and rhythm bands, folk dancing (including wheelchair dancing), talent shows, indoor and outdoor gardening, cooking, arts and crafts, bingo, movies, current events discussions, planning and writing a monthly newsletter, library activities, and games such as cards, checkers, chess, and a host of others.

Forms of recreation for disoriented patients are considerably more difficult to plan and conduct but equally essential. Senile or otherwise confused patients respond well to sensory stimuli. Music plays an effectual role, and frequently the elderly patient seems charged with new life when he listens to songs he knew when he was young. Occasionally his reaction is to cry, but these are tears to be welcomed. They mean that he's responding, that he's experiencing emotion and recall. Storytelling appeals to some disoriented patients, although others lose interest quickly. Homemade scrapbooks (that can be put together by alert patients) provide hours of diversion when they are composed of large brightly colored pictures of familiar sights such as houses, cars, trees, gardens, children playing, and easily recognizable family scenes and situations. These pictures can be cut from old magazines. The sense of touch provides disoriented patients with satisfaction in fingering objects of diversified sizes, shapes, and textures. Scrapbooks can be comprised of ribbons of velvet, satin, and grosgrain; small shells of different shapes and textures; buttons that vary from rough to smooth, from square to round, and from small to large; and pieces of lace, velvet, corduroy, and satin. Color plays a significant part in these, doubling the appeal to the senses.

Activities must be provided for the bedridden: reading, sewing, compiling scrapbooks, collecting items such as stamps or coins, painting, making holiday decorations and writing for the newspaper. Passive recreation can be accomplished through a piano on the nursing floor and a volunteer to play and perhaps sing, a record player, reading aloud, and word games.

Trips outside of the nursing home are invigorating and memorable for patients who have medical permission to leave the premises. The dreary routine of confinement is alleviated by excursions to museums, movies, theaters, concerts, or the zoo; short shopping expeditions; regular visits to local Golden Age groups; leisurely rides through the countryside to enjoy the autumn or spring foliage; boat day trips and similar outings. The most handicapped and most disoriented patients enjoy outdoor picnics and barbecues, even if these are held on limited areas of the lawn or terrace. Bringing the community *into* the nursing home has value, too. This can be done by inviting community groups to hold their meetings within the nursing home and by enlisting volunteers from the community, thus giving evidence to the patients that society remembers and cares.

Recreation frequently augments rehabilitation therapies. Simple question and answer games or sing-alongs can be gainful for the patients in speech therapy. Tossing a beach ball or playing darts, for instance, can add immeasurably to the efforts of the occupational and physical therapists who are working to develop coordination of muscles in the arms and hands.

Calendars of recreational activities for a full week, clearly printed on large colorful posters, should be placed in the lobby, dining room, dayrooms, and other strategic areas so that all patients can elect which activities they care to join. Optimally, recreation programs should be provided seven days a week and should cover at least several evenings.

The Recreation Director

The recreation director, sometimes referred to as the activities leader, has the responsibility for developing, scheduling, and conducting a multifaceted program geared to meet the social and diversional needs of alert, disoriented, and bedridden patients. She is directly responsible to the administrator (and to the consultant when there is one on staff) and works closely with the nursing department and with the physical, occupational, and speech therapists.

Nurses and attending physicians must be kept aware of how and what their patients are doing in recreation since this is an integral aspect of restorative care. Thus the recreation director is obligated to make regular entries in the patients' medical charts and frequently on their patient-care plans.

Religious Needs. The recreation director has the added responsibility of providing for the patients' spiritual needs. She recruits clergymen in the predominant faiths and, with their cooperation, schedules regular religious services in the home. Any of these services should be open to patients of all faiths, although none should be forced to attend. The recreation director makes arrangements for handicapped patients to be escorted to and from formal services, either by volunteers or by aides or orderlies designated by charge nurses. When arrangements cannot be made to hold religious services within the nursing home, it is incumbent upon the recreation director to assist the administrator in setting up procedures that allow medically qualified patients to be driven to neighborhood churches. Provision of the necessary cars or bus would then be the obligation of the nursing home. Clergymen should be regularly available to the patients on an individual basis for counseling, encouragement, or the fulfillment of spiritual need.

You may want to ask how frequently services are held in the

religion of your patient's faith, and how often the religious leader comes to visit patients individually. Ask either the administrator or the recreation director and expect an easy and straightforward answer.

Volunteers. In a small or medium-sized nursing home the recreation director serves also as director of volunteers. The larger nursing home may employ a volunteer director charged with that single responsibility. Volunteers must be recruited, oriented, assigned, trained, and supervised to assist in the recreation department so that it is not limited to the minimal number of programs that can be conducted by the recreation director alone. Volunteers also supplement nursing services and provide personal assistance to patients in tasks such as writing letters, reading aloud, and what is termed "friendly visiting," a matter of talking with patients and listening to what they have to say but withholding personal opinion or advice. Most volunteers serve in recreation and nursing programs, but many work in other departments of the home.

As a rule many community resources and many areas for volunteer service are left untapped. The local department of education may cooperate by sending in teachers or student teachers who can help the younger patients continue their education and assist others with overcoming language barriers or pursuing fields of special interest. Librarians can be asked to teach patients to run their own library; a handful of reporters may be willing to come in to report on news events; professional photographers can assist amateurs; the local congressman may welcome the opportunity to address the patients on new developments in health legislation. After all, these same patients will cast absentee ballots in November. And, perhaps most important of all, the patients themselves can volunteer in numerous capacities and enjoy the same self-satisfaction and recognition that are earned by community volunteers.

Evaluating the Recreation Department. The most revealing

indication of whether or not a recreation program is success-fully planned and administered is the number of patients who participate and the number who sit idly in their bedrooms or in corridors or dayrooms. I can think of few sights more in-tolerable than wheelchairs lined against a wall and the patients sitting in them staring into space. There can be no clearer manifestation of an inadequate and thoughtless recreation pro-gram, unless—far worse—it is evidence of medical policy to keep patients quiet and undemanding through overuse of tranquiliz-ing medications.

A simple evaluation tool is the recreation calendar. If you don't find one posted in the lobby or in the patients' areas, or even if you do, ask to see several, covering different dates. One is not enough, because hopefully there is variance from week to week.

Observe a number of recreational activities firsthand. In-quire of the charge nurse if the recreation director enters regu-lar notations on the patients' medical charts and patient-care plans. By all means ask the patients what they think of the recreation program and how frequently they participate. If they participate seldom or not at all, ask them their reasons.

Rehabilitation Therapy

Rehabilitation therapy is a medically prescribed and pro-fessionally administered curative process. *Occupational ther-apy* refers to medically prescribed professional treatment de-signed to improve the muscular coordination of hands and arms (the upper extremities) and eye-hand coordination and is acccomplished by means of occupational exercise. *Physical therapy* refers to medically prescribed professional treatment of upper and lower extremities through the use of physical media. *Speech therapy* makes use of speech as a tool toward alleviating speech impediment and also in the treatment of aphasia. Aphasia is a frequent aftermath of stroke (cerebral vascular accident, or CVA) and involves not only the inability of its victim to express himself in words, but often the further tragedy of partial or even total loss of verbal comprehension, written as well as oral.

These three therapies are commonly offered in skilled nursing facilities. If any one of them is not available on the premises of the nursing home, arrangements must be made with qualified resources outside of the home (for which the nursing facility assumes professional and administrative responsibility) or patients requiring this care cannot be admitted.

A friend of mine placed her father in a nursing home a number of years ago. He was the victim of a stroke that had claimed the use of his left side and his power of speech, and he died after several months in the facility. During the course of his stay my friend had been delighted with the nursing care and the atmosphere of the home. She didn't realize until long after her father's death that he should have been given speech therapy on a regular basis. The home had no arrangements for speech therapy and made no mention of it. Either her father's attending physician had been guilty of failure to prescribe speech therapy or the nursing home had admitted him illegally.

The therapists' contribution to the total rehabilitation of the patient is achieved through accurate interpretation and administration of the attending physician's written prescriptions and is directed at restoring the patient to self-maintenance. Patients are scheduled for specified regular sessions, which, barring emergency, they are required to attend.

The patient's progress is reviewed regularly by the attending physician and the therapists and is reevaluated at maximum intervals of thirty days. Records of reviews, evaluations, and treatment plans are incorporated into the patient's medical chart.

The therapists have a dual responsibility to the administrator and the medical director; they work closely with each other and with the nursing and recreation departments. Practice is restricted to professionals, who are qualified through experience and postgraduate training, and to qualified assistants working under the direct supervision of professionals.

Physicians frequently prescribe "Instruction in ADL" (activities of daily living) although this can be carried through without medical prescription. The appropriate therapist evaluates the patient and outlines a course of treatment, which is brought back to the physician for his final determination. However, the full potential of this training can be realized only when the therapist educates the nursing staff to supplement the therapeutic process. When the physical therapist trains a patient in relearning how to walk, for instance, these sessions are usually scheduled for fifteen- or twenty-minute intervals, perhaps on a daily basis or perhaps three times a week. Progress is bound to be minimal unless aides and orderlies complement the efforts of the therapist by assisting the patient in regular daily ambulation. Similarly, tasks that are within the realm of the occupational therapist—combing hair, shaving, washing, and dressing —must be practiced routinely if the patient is to gain significant headway. All of the nursing staff, who should be well indoctrinated in the goals and methods of restorative nursing and trained by the therapists in procedures for rehabilitation, serve as assistants to the speech therapist just by making it a daily routine to talk with their patients. They reinforce this assistance by making it a point to speak slowly, enunciate carefully, repeat the patient's name, deliberately refer to surrounding objects, and so forth. The supplemental capacity of recreation is discussed on page 78.

Therapists play a significant role in discharge planning. They confer with medical, nursing, and social services in order to help make the best possible provision for the patient's placement after discharge from the facility: return to home, sharing a residence with family members or friends, intermediate care facility, senior citizens residence, or possibly home-health or out-patient hospital care for the continuance of treatment. One of the factors determining whether or not a patient will be able to live alone is the measure of his independence in the activities of daily living.

Occupational Therapy

Occupational therapy devotes its treatments to the development of the fine muscles of the hands and arms. It is less concerned with strength than with coordination.

The therapy is often confused by the layman with the arts and crafts program in recreation. Were you to observe a group of patients working with paints, clay, or wood in occupational therapy, you might well conclude that these are just about the same things that others are doing in recreation. Medical objective and precision are the factors that differentiate the two.

The area for occupational therapy should be separate and apart from recreation. Preferably, the room should be spacious, light, and pleasant. The kinds of equipment you can expect to see in a well-furbished setting are large worktables, a sewing machine, ironing board and iron, kiln, looms for rug-making, a typewriter, scraps of leather, hanks of wool and both knitting and crocheting needles, scissors and needles and thread, paints and canvases, clay, tiles, wood, sandpaper, handsaws, hammers, screwdrivers, paste and an assortment of boxes, bottles, candles, colored paper and the like for making small ornamental gifts. Many more items of similar nature may enhance the potential of the departmental goals; on the other hand, there may be fewer.

Every well-equipped occupational therapy department has a selection of functional devices designed to help patients relearn the ordinary activities of daily living: special implements for eating, for combing or brushing hair, for closing buttons and zippers, putting on shoes, and similar daily routines.

An occasional nursing home goes so far as to install a kitchen area where working surfaces can be easily reached by wheelchair patients. This provides many women with occupational therapy in its purest sense, assisting them to relearn the simple tasks that once played an important role in their lives and hopefully may have equal meaning to them in the future.

It is the policy of many nursing homes to exhibit articles made by the patients in occupational therapy or in arts and crafts programs. Usually these exhibits are set up in glass-enclosed cases in the front lobby, and, from time to time, a day —or a week—is set aside for the sale of these objets d'art, with one or more patients in charge. Monies realized are used either to purchase working materials or for a patient outing or party voted upon by the contributing patients.

Physical Therapy

Physical therapy devotes itself to the development and coordination of the gross muscles in arms, hands, legs, feet, back, neck, and most of the body; training in the use of prosthetic limbs; and adeptness with crutches, canes, and walkers.

The physical therapy room must include equipment such as parallel bars with a full-length mirror placed so that patients can observe their mistakes as well as their progress, corner stairs, rope pulleys for strengthening arm muscles, exercycles for strengthening leg muscles, hydrocollator hot packs, heat lamps, whirlpool bath, electrotherapy and diathermy accouterments, crutches, canes, and walkers, and many other devices. Physical therapy employs a wide range of physical agents other than drugs, including "light, heat, cold, water, and electricity, or . . . mechanical apparatus."[1]

The physical therapy department is actively involved with training patients—and educating nursing staff to augment the training—in activities of daily living such as walking, climbing stairs, moving from bed to wheelchair to toilet, raising arms, and numerous other activities involving the use and coordination of large muscles. It concerns itself also with teaching safety measures to the nursing staff for lifting and turning patients, safety for both the patients and the staff members.

[1] *Dorland's Illustrated Medical Dictionary*, 24th ed., W. B. Saunders Company, Philadelphia, 1965.

Speech Therapy and Audiology

The primary function of speech therapy in a nursing home is to help aphasic patients relearn the meaning and the use of words. This training applies to the written word almost as frequently as it does to the oral. Aphasia implies loss of the ability to communicate through words, but it can also mean that the patient can hear the spoken word yet have no idea of its meaning; and that the patient can read a familiar word or, rather, look at it but have no idea of its meaning.

It's an interesting sidelight that frequently an aphasic patient can be helped back to the use and understanding of speech by reverting to the language of his early childhood. The patient who came to this country from Italy at the age of 6, and who has spoken English for the past seventy-five years, may well respond to the Italian language rather than English. In such an instance, his family and friends who are versed in the first language he ever knew can approximate the role of the speech therapist.

The speech therapist uses a number of relatively simple tools, but her own patience and perspicacity must be highly developed. Equipment for speech therapy includes a blackboard and chalk, fairly large colorful posters illustrating familiar objects such as a car, for instance, and underneath the picture the word C A R printed in bold letters; numerous sheets of drawing paper with large or easily held crayons or colored pencils; and usually tape and a tape recorder so that the patient can listen to his own speech patterns.

Usually the speech therapist is equipped with an audiometer to test hearing. If she finds that there is a hearing loss, she refers the matter to the patient's attending physician, who, in turn, refers the patient to a hearing specialist.

Sometimes a small room is set aside for the purpose of speech therapy and audiology. More frequently, however, speech therapy is administered in any unoccupied quiet area—perhaps the beauty parlor on a day that it's closed, the dining room during midmorning or midafternoon, a vacant office, or the patient's bedside. Noise and other distractions constitute serious deterrents to effective speech therapy and certainly to the testing of hearing.

Evaluating the Rehabilitation Therapies. Assuming that you are neither a physician nor a professional in the field of rehabilitation, you will have only two yardsticks for measuring the performance of the rehabilitation therapies. Do the patients seem contented and is the atmosphere warm and friendly? Is your patient's attending physician satisfied with both the goals and the achievements of the therapies? Do *not* judge the efficacy of the department by whether or not your patient improves in function. It may well be that the only practical and medically prescribed goal for your patient is the maintenance of his present level of activity or even the retardation of inevitable further deterioration.

Social Service

The goal of social service is to identify medically related social and emotional needs of patients and provide the services necessary to meet them. Social service begins with the patient's admission to the facility, or sometimes earlier with a pre-admission interview, and concludes only when the patient is discharged.

Sometimes a large voluntary (nonprofit) nursing home has a well-staffed social service department with some workers assigned to specific caseloads and others to intake interviews and assessments. This is the exception rather than the rule. Generally a nursing home designates one staff member to the role of social service worker, either on a full-time or part-time basis. If the employee is not a qualified social service worker, regular consultation must be provided by either a qualified social service worker or a recognized social agency. Federal standards call for "sufficient supportive personnel" to meet the patients' needs and "adequate" facilities for the personnel to ensure privacy for interviews and easy accessibility for both patients and staff. If the nursing home does not provide social services on the premises, arrangements are made to refer patients to appropriate social agencies.

All records are classified as strictly confidential. They cover personal and family problems relating to the patient's illness and care and other pertinent social data. If a patient is referred to an outside resource, records are maintained of such referrals. These are incorporated into the patient's medical record.

The social service worker deals directly with the patient in helping him to cope with emotional problems arising from his health status and his institutionalization. Frequently it is necessary to work with relatives as well as with patients.

The emotional problem most frequently met by nursing-home patients is the difficulty of adaptation to unnatural surroundings and unnatural living. Perhaps the patient has had his own room for the past ten years or shared his room only with a beloved wife. Now he's living in a two-bedded or a four-bedded room, and he can't adjust to the lack of privacy. One patient's snoring keeps him awake at night, another's incessant talking deprives him of quiet times to read or think or rest, or the patient in the next bed objects to his habit of reading into the wee hours. He wants to get well and be released from the confines of the nursing home; he willingly cooperates with the doctor, the nurses, the therapists, and the technicians, but he cannot adjust to the total annihilation of privacy. This is typical of the kind of difficulty that falls into the realm of social service. Handling the problem can be simple or complex. It depends on the patient and his background and his own emotional potential.

On occasion the social service worker bypasses the patient and works exclusively with his relative, as the case of Mrs.

Lewis illustrates. Mrs. Lewis was a patient of 83, completely senile and totally dependent on the home and its staff for her every need. Her son, a married man of about sixty, came to visit her every evening on his way home from work. It was his custom to arrive at about six o'clock, just after the supper trays had been removed. Every evening Mrs. Lewis greeted him by saying, "Son, they didn't give me any supper tonight. Nothing at all." Every evening he went to the charge nurse who assured him that his mother had eaten and eaten well. Mrs. Lewis remained so adamant and so persistent in her protestations that finally her son went to the social service worker, Mrs. Dickinson. She promised to look into the matter for him and report back just as soon as she had determined what was going on. In a few days Mrs. Dickinson telephoned Mr. Lewis at work and asked him to arrange to visit his mother a little earlier, at five o'clock instead of at six. Mr. Lewis arrived promptly at five, and supper was served to his mother about fifteen minutes later. She ate every mouthful that was offered to her and apparently enjoyed it thoroughly. Then an aide removed her tray. No sooner had the aide left her bedside than Mrs. Lewis looked up at her son and said, "They didn't give me any supper tonight. Nothing at all."

This was a problem rightfully directed to the social service worker, who was not involved either with the dietary department that provided the meals or with the nursing department that served them. Dietary or nursing personnel could have been defensive, could have covered up for negligence. Social service was impartial and tactful in its investigation; the mystery was easily unfolded, and the son was relieved of a worry that had been gnawing at him for several weeks.

Sometimes the social service worker must handle a problem by dealing with both the patient and the relative. Laura Simpson was a 28-year-old victim of amytrophic lateral sclerosis, more commonly known as Lou Gehrig's disease. She was confined to a wheelchair, unable to feed or toilet or dress herself, unable to propel her own wheelchair, and unable to speak clearly. She was probably the most unhappy young woman I have ever known. In addition to the nearly unbearable burden of her physical deterioration, she had been all but abandoned by her mother and sister. Her father was dead, and her mother had remarried about two years before Laura was institutionalized. Her only sister was healthy, attractive, and happily married with two children of her own. Mother and sister came to see Laura three or perhaps four times during the course of a year, although both lived in the neighboring county. Always they came together, as though fortified by one another. Whether it was an inability to face Laura in her present disfigured condition, feelings of guilt, or total indifference on their part, the end result was that Laura grieved. She wept openly for them, and on weekends and holidays that lured most visitors into the home, she had frequent temper tantrums and wailed that her family never came to see her.

The social service worker was contacted by the nursing staff. He worked with Laura to help her to understand that her mother and sister had never stopped loving her, but that they were unable to cope with the reality of her illness. He worked with Laura's mother in an effort to make her see that her second marriage would not be jeopardized if she gave more time and thought to Laura; and he tried to get through to her sister in an attempt to make her realize that her world was not limited to her new family, but still included Laura. This was a long, arduous task. The social worker was just beginning to make headway when one night Laura's breathing muscles failed her, and she died within minutes.

Patients' personal financial problems related to their illness and institutionalization also come to the attention of the social service worker but are a great deal easier to handle. Here are direct routes to travel. A patient may be admitted as private-paying and, after a while, exhaust his funds. Then the social service worker assists him with completing forms to apply for Medicaid coverage. Sometimes it happens that a patient has been on welfare before his admission to the nursing home. During his stay his bills are paid by Medicaid. As he approaches the date of discharge his welfare funds must be restored to him so that he will have monies after he is no longer institutionalized. The social worker is charged with the responsibility of contacting the Department of Social Services and making the necessary arrangements for the patient to be reinstated on the welfare rolls.

When a patient is to be discharged from the nursing home, his attending physician decides whether he can return to living alone or with family or friends or if he needs to be transferred to an intermediate care facility, senior citizens residence, or other institution. In making his final decision the physician will confer with members of the nursing staff and with rehabilitation therapists, and will rely to a large extent on the discharge plan and on the information that has been regularly entered into the patient's medical record. Sociomedical information specified by the social service worker provides an important resource for determining whether or not the patient is able to return to his former living arrangements. If the patient is to be discharged to another institution that provides a different level of care, it behooves the social worker to find a bed in an appropriate facility, hopefully one that is located conveniently for regular visits of family and friends.

Every social worker plays a cooperative role with medical, nursing, dietary, recreation and rehabilitation services, as well as with the business office that maintains current records of patients' financial circumstances. Medically related problems of the patients invariably involve a number of disciplines. Every staff member requires the joint efforts of every other staff member; and nowhere is this more true than with social services.

Evaluating Social Service. Unless you or your patient has occasion to make use of the home's social service, there is no way for you to evaluate its effectiveness firsthand. Ask your patient's attending physician for his estimate; and from there address a good many more questions to the medical director or to the administrator.

Are social services available within the home? If not, what

agencies are used and how are patients transported? If so, is the social worker qualified or does he work under the general supervision of a consultant? How much time does the consultant give? Is the social worker part time or full time? If he is part time, how many hours a week are involved? Does he have other duties in the home? What are the other duties?

I suggest this line of questioning because I know of a nursing home that squeaked through by meeting the letter of the law but hardly its intent. A qualified social service worker came to the home three hours a week in the role of consultant. The administrator's secretary was given the title of part-time social worker. The secretary was intelligent and empathetic with the patients' needs. Nevertheless, the appointment to her new role (which brought with it a small raise in salary) was pure fiasco. Her time was heavily occupied as the administrator's secretary, and the most she could do by way of social service was to manage a few minutes with patients who came to her desk to ask for help. Actually she served as henchman to the social service consultant by reporting to him whatever problems were brought to her attention. She had neither the time nor the background to be instrumental in their solution; and obviously the consultant could do little with three hours a week to devote to a patient population of almost two hundred.

If you think that your patient or you will need the help of social service, then be sure to avoid this sort of pitfall. And, in any event, recognize it as a lack of concern for the personal needs of the patients.

ERRATUM

On page 93, line 4 should read:
Medicare once a patient has reached 65 years of age) , (2) Medi-

7

Meeting the Costs of Care

THERE ARE AT LEAST SEVEN different means of meeting the costs of a nursing-home confinement: (1) health insurance coverage with a private company (generally designed to supplement Medicare and Medicaid together, (6) hospital-skilled nursing care, Part A, (3) Medicare, Parts A and B, (4) Medicaid, (5) Medicare and Medicaid together, (6) hospital-skilled nursing facility contract based on Blue Cross benefits, and (7) private direct payment. Frequently costs are met by combinations of the above: a patient uses up Medicare benefits and then pays privately; another patient first pays privately, exhausts his funds, and then applies for Medicaid, etc.

Private Insurance

Any insurance company policy providing benefits in a nursing home will be an individual one and will present its own details of what to expect by way of coverage. There is no practical way of discussing such policies here since they are both numerous and varied and offer unique terms. However, two facts pertain to such policies in relation to Medicare and Medicaid recipients. All appropriate benefits of a privately-owned policy must be applied to nursing-home and medical costs before Medicare funds can be tapped. If your patient qualifies for Medicaid benefits, he must report the ownership of such a policy, and the local Medicaid office is charged with the decision of whether or not the policy should be maintained.

Medicare and Medicaid: Similarities and Differences

In the pages that follow, I will present a brief outline of the structure and purpose of Medicare and Medicaid, eligibility requirements for each, and the benefits they offer to patients in nursing homes. Both programs offer a wide range of benefits in almost every area of medical and medically related care, but I'm concerned here only with their application to patients in skilled nursing facilities.

Medicare (Title XVIII of the Social Security Act) and Medicaid (Title XIX) were both enacted in 1965 as amendments to the Social Security Act. Medicare was first implemented for skilled nursing care, then known as extended care, in January 1967[1] Medicaid became effective for nursing facilities in January 1966, although at that time coverage was effective in only six states and in Puerto Rico.[2] At first substantially higher standards were mandated for providers of Medicare than for providers of Medicaid. It was only in 1973 that requirements for the two became identical. Now a skilled nursing facility that qualifies for one program automatically qualifies for the other, and patients who are covered by Medicaid can expect

[1] *Medicare: Health Insurance for the Aged, 1967, Section 3.3: Participating Extended Care Facilities,* U.S., SSA, ORS, Washington, D.C., 1971.

[2] *Characteristics of State Medical Assistance Programs Under Title XIX of the Social Security Act,* U.S., DHEW, SRS, Public Assistance Series Number 49: 1970 Edition, Washington, D.C., 1971.

the same standards of nursing-home care as can the recipients of Medicare.

Medicare is a federally administered compulsory insurance program for the aged. It offers all insured persons identical benefits (and restrictions) whether in Massachusetts or in Guam. Coverage is available in all fifty states, the District of Columbia, Guam, Puerto Rico, the Virgin Islands, and American Samoa.

Enrollment is not limited to citizens only, but extends to everyone over 65 who has paid into social security for a minimum period of twenty quarters, not necessarily consecutive, and to federal employees who pay into a retirement plan other than social security. (Some railroad retirees are ineligible because of other insurance plans.) Medicare is also available to persons of any age who have been receiving social security disability benefits for a minimum period of twenty-four consecutive months (and, in a hospital setting, to victims of kidney disease who require dialysis). Under any of these conditions, enrollment in the Medicare program is available to people of all income brackets, whether multimillionaires or recipients of welfare funds. Application for Medicare benefits should be made to the local social security office, usually about three months before reaching the age of 65.

Medicaid is a program of financial assistance offered at the option of individual states to numerous persons who cannot pay the full costs of medical care. The program is state-administered but subject to federal guidelines. Federal taxes subsidize a minimum of 50 percent of costs and a maximum (at present) of 83 percent, depending on the average per capita income of the individual state. The difference in cost is picked up either entirely by state taxes or sometimes by a combination of state and county taxes. The responsible state is that in which the health care facility is located; the responsible county is that of the patient's last legal residence.

Medicaid programs operate in all fifty states, the District of Columbia, Guam, Puerto Rico, and the Virgin Islands. Because the program is state-administered and exists at the option of the state, eligibility requirements and benefits vary accordingly. Application for Medicaid benefits should be made to the local social service or welfare department.

Civil Rights. Both Medicare and Medicaid programs are subject to Title VI of the Civil Rights Act, which states that "No person in the United States shall, on the ground of race, color, or national origin, be excluded from participation in, be denied the benefit of, or be subjected to discrimination under any program or activity receiving Federal financial assistance." If there is any question of discrimination being practiced in the nursing home, report it immediately to the local social security office (for Medicare), the social services or welfare office (for Medicaid), or directly to the U.S. Department of Health, Education and Welfare in Washington, D.C. Bear in mind, however, that the nursing home that restricts admissions to private-paying patients is not bound by the Civil Rights Act since it is not accepting federal financial assistance. Therefore it can limit its patient population to one religion, one color, one nationality, one disease, one handicap—one anything.

Medicare, Part A

Eligibility and Benefits

The coverage of Part A of Medicare, otherwise known as hospital insurance, extends also to skilled nursing facilities (formerly termed extended care facilities). This part of Medicare insurance is available *at no cost* to everyone who qualifies, as explained on page 95. It is subsidized through regular payroll deductions for social security, matched by employees and employers, and submitted independently by the self-employed.

If your patient is enrolled in the Medicare program, Part A can pay for most of the costs in a skilled nursing facility during a limited period of time. This holds true, however, *only* if your patient has been hospitalized for a minimum of three days and has been discharged from the hospital within a fourteen-day period prior to admission to the nursing home; if his physician prescribes this level of care because of continued need for daily skilled nursing or rehabilitation therapy; and if the admitting diagnosis to the nursing home is the same as the original admitting diagnosis to the hospital. All of these conditions must be met in order to qualify for Medicare coverage in a skilled nursing facility. If it happens that your patient is discharged from a skilled nursing facility but is readmitted to the same or another one within fourteen days, he can continue to use his Medicare coverage providing that he still requires that level of care and providing, of course, that he has not used up his benefits.

Medicare makes payments directly to the nursing facility through a fiscal intermediary, a health insurance organization appointed by the social security administration. It will pay for up to a maximum of one hundred days of care for each "spell of illness" in a skilled nursing facility. The spell of illness, often referred to as the benefit period, ends sixty days after discharge from the facility. A new benefit period or new spell of illness begins any time after this sixty-day period, provided that the patient is again hospitalized for a minimum of three consecutive days and again meets all the basic requirements.

Limitations of Medicare Coverage, Part A

Do *not* anticipate that Medicare will cover the total costs of a hundred days in any one benefit period. It won't cover all the costs, and it very well may not cover the hundred days.

To begin with, Medicare will pay full per-diem costs for a maximum of the first twenty days only, provided that all twenty are medically approved. Your patient will have to contribute to the daily charges of any of the following eighty days that may be medically approved for his continued stay. Originally the patient's share was $5 per diem; at present writing it is $9. By the time you read these words, it may be higher.

Using the $9 figure, you might assume that if your patient is covered by Part A of Medicare, and if he remains in the skilled nursing facility for one hundred days, then the most his care can cost him is $720 (80 days multiplied by $9). Don't make this assumption.

Part A of Medicare will pay for a bed in a two- or four-bedded room (or a private room if it is medically essential); all meals including a special diet; regular nursing services; physical, occupational, and speech therapy (when they are included in the nursing home's per diem rate); and drugs, appliances, equipment, and services that are customarily covered by the nursing home's daily rate.

Part A will not cover any physician services or private-duty nurses under any circumstances, and it will not cover extra charges for a private room unless it is medically prescribed. In no event does coverage extend to custodial care or to a level of care that demands less than daily skilled nursing, rehabilitation therapy, or both. And, of course, it never extends to convenience items such as personal telephone, radio, television, or services of barber or beautician.

Further, and of greater impact, Medicare may discontinue your patient's benefits after a period of ten days, or thirty, or umpteen. Payment is discontinued if, *at any time,* it is medically considered that your patient's condition no longer requires the level of professional care for which he was admitted. The utilization review committee (Chapter 8) periodically reviews your patient's health status, the care he is being given, and the care he requires, as do his attending physician, the intermediary organization that works with both Medicare and the facility, and the Medical Review Team discussed on pages 109 and 110. If it is medically determined that the progress of your patient indicates that he now needs a lesser level of care,

Medicare payments are discontinued within three days. You—or he—should be given immediate and written notification of this decision.

Occasionally the medical staff of the health insurance intermediary or the Medical Review Team will decide that a patient's benefits should have been discontinued at a date prior to the determining review. In such an event, his benefits are canceled retroactively, and he is personally billed by the nursing home for costs incurred subsequent to the cutoff date. If he is unable to make payment, he can then apply for Medicaid assistance. This will be granted if he is financially and medically qualified in accordance with the provisions of the state.

Abrupt and unexpected cancellation of Medicare benefits can be a traumatic turn of events for patient and relative alike. There are two contradictory aspects to this action: one to be understood and the other to be deplored. The first is the practical necessity of economics: to purchase essential services but to eliminate or at least curtail the nonessential. Frequently, as a Medicare patient progresses in health status, a schedule of less intensive care can meet all his health needs at a lower cost to government and taxpayers. An intermediate health-care facility or a home-health program or perhaps the family can take over successfully. Most of us are directly affected by Medicare funding through social security taxes. Cautious allotment of these funds can keep Medicare overhead at a reasonable minimum and channel the total purchasing power to fill genuine need.

Less understandable is the Medicare procedure for evaluating the level of professional care required by an individual patient. When this is determined by the intermediary's medical staff, judgment is based on pen and paper reports submitted at regular intervals by the nursing facility. Reports are made on routine printed forms. A licensed nurse submits requested specific information gathered from the patient's medical record and enters in the limited space provided a few words of professional comments on the patient's overall condition. There is the old maxim of one picture being worth a thousand words.

In this instance one direct patient medical examination might well outweigh a lexicon.

Two factors soften the blow of unanticipated and sudden disallowance of further Medicare-reimbursed institutionalization. First, there exists a procedure for contesting the cancellation of Medicare benefits. The procedure is unwieldy and time-consuming, but on occasion it can prove fruitful. Your local social security office can help you to launch such action if you feel it is called for. Second, and more generally applicable, is the process of discharge planning, which is originated within the first few days of the patient's admission and continued throughout his stay. The medical-nursing-rehabilitation-social service team works consistently toward planning the most practical and effective placement for the patient when he no longer requires skilled nursing. Thus, if your patient's benefits are unexpectedly terminated, you can at least look to the road that has been mapped for him to travel.

Professional Standards Review Organizations (PSRO's)

A promising turn of events appears likely with the advent of Professional Standards Review Organizations (PSRO's). The idea of peer review was initiated by the American Medical Association, and subsequently expanded and strengthened under the leadership of Republican Senator Wallace F. Bennett of Utah. In its fuller, more comprehensive form, it was signed into law in October 1972 as an amendment to the Social Security Act. We now stand at the threshold of this new program, with numerous aspects still to be effected before the legislation becomes a functioning reality.

The review process by PSRO's provides for professional (physician) review of the quality and utilization of Medicare- and Medicaid-reimbursed health programs and the appropriateness of admissions; and should one day expand to cover quality and utilization of services for private-paying patients. The concept of the PSRO is founded on the premise that physicians are the only persons qualified to determine the necessity of services prescribed by other physicians, that the utilization review process (Chapter 8) is frequently a token mechanism, and that therefore "Peer review should be performed at the local level with professional [nonprofit] societies acting as sponsors and supervisors.[3] Professionally established norms of care are to be used as "review checkpoints" but not as definitive data for determination of duration of stay.

As of May 1974, 131 nonprofit professional associations composed of licensed physicians (medical societies, health-care foundations, medical foundations, medical institutes, health councils, etc.) representing forty-six states, the District of Columbia, and Puerto Rico had applied either for status as conditional PSRO's (there is a two-year conditional approval period) or as statewide resource centers; or they had applied for funds for establishing PSRO's or for further developing standards. It is proposed that Statewide Professional Standards Review Councils and a National Professional Standards Review Council shall serve in advisory capacities to the individual PSRO's.

Medical reviews to be made by the Professional Standards Review Organizations are presently scheduled for only "periodic" or "regular" intervals. However, there is every likelihood that time and collective experience will bring about numerous specifications dictated by findings and by costs.

The programs will be financed through federal funding. The control of government financed health care should offset the new expenditure. PSRO determination that a patient no longer warrants skilled nursing care will be cause for cancellation of Medicare and/or Medicaid benefits and will in no way eliminate this contingency.

It is to be hoped that the new procedure will benefit long-

[3] *Background Material Relating to Professional Standards Review Organizations,* Committee on Finance, U.S. Senate, U.S. Government Printing Office, Washington, D.C., 1974.

term patients through tightening the utilization review process, providing personal and objective medical assessment in determining duration of stay, submitting disciplinary recommendations to curtail unwarranted patient stay, and by "monitoring underservicing as well as overutilization of services."[4]

Medicare, Part B

Part B of Medicare is a medical insurance program that helps to defray the costs of many medical services including a number that are provided in skilled nursing facilities. The program is optional and is available to all those who are enrolled in Part A of Medicare.

Contrary to Part A, there is a cost to the consumer for enrolling in Part B. As of this writing, the cost is $6.70 a month to the insured and is met by an equal payment of $6.70 a month by the federal government. In 1967 this cost was $3 monthly; in 1973 it was $5.80, so again further increases may be imminent. However, the law now states that increases in the consumer's share of payment for this medical coverage can be effected only if there has been a general increase in social security cash benefits subsequent to the previous increase in premium. Thus it is possible that in the future the federal government may become responsible for more than half the costs.

Part B coverage is automatically given to every recipient of Part A unless he specifically requests otherwise. If he receives social security checks, whether pension or disability income, the monthly premium charges are deducted. If he receives none of these monthly checks, he may pay his monthly premium directly; or, in some instances, the cost is picked up by a state assistance program. If an individual elects not to be covered when he is first eligible and decides to enroll at some future

[4] From a speech by Senator Wallace F. Bennett.

date, the monthly premium is slightly higher, depending on the time interval that has elapsed.

The monthly premium entitles the consumer to the equivalent of a major medical insurance policy that pays 80 percent of all reasonable medical charges after a basic deductible of $60 in any calendar year. Sometimes medical expenses incurred during the last three months of a calendar year can be applied toward the $60 deductible for the following year. If this provision can prove beneficial to your patient, contact your local social security office for further details. X-ray and laboratory charges in a skilled nursing facility (or a hospital) are paid in full and do not contribute to the deductible.

Policy coverage includes medical and surgical services by a doctor of medicine or osteopathy. This means that the monthly visits of your patient's attending physician fall into the category of covered services, as do some of his possible emergency visits—those that are approved by Medicare as meeting genuine emergency. Also included are diagnostic tests and procedures, medical supplies, drugs and biologicals, dental surgery, and some services of podiatrists and chiropractors. Ambulance service is covered when transportation by other means would be hazardous to the patient's health and when the patient is taken to the nearest facility that provides the appropriate level of care. If the patient chooses a facility located at a greater distance, he will have to personally assume the costs of the additional mileage.

When further stay in a nursing home is disapproved before the end of a benefit period, this decision automatically cancels all Medicare benefits (Parts A and B) for any continued confinement in the facility. Sometimes, however, it's decided that the patient requires skilled nursing, but that his physical therapy treatments, for instance, are no longer effective and therefore are to be terminated. Many nursing homes include physical and occupational therapy as part of their daily rates, and they are thus covered by Part A of Medicare. Many other homes charge separately for these therapeutic services, and Medicare patients must then look to Part B for coverage. If it is the determination of the attending physician, the utilization review committee, the intermediary's medical team, or the PSRO Medical Review Team that the patient can remain in the nursing home as a Medicare patient, but that he no longer requires physical therapy, Part A may continue per diem payment, but Part B will discontinue any reimbursement for physical therapy.

Further Medicare Information

The hospital's medical social service worker or the nursing facility's administrator, admissions officer, or social worker can probably answer any questions you may have or provide any technical assistance you may need. Sometimes the physician is accurate in his knowledge of both Medicare and Medicaid, but frequently he shares the same areas of confusion as the general public.

All questions relative to Medicare—eligibility requirements, benefits, restrictions, costs, and enrollment period—can be brought directly to your local social security office for accurate up-to-date information. Meanwhile, contact that office for the free booklet issued by the Department of Health, Education and Welfare entitled *Your Medicare Handbook*. This is a comprehensive and tersely written account of just about everything you may want to know about Parts A and B of Medicare.

Supplemental Security Income (SSI)

Another pamphlet you may want to have on hand is entitled *Introducing Supplemental Security Income*. This can be obtained from the Department of Health, Education and Welfare in Washington, D.C., or from your local social security or welfare office.

The Supplemental Security Income program was put into effect on January 1, 1974, and replaces the former public assistance programs to the aged, blind, disabled, and indigent (except in the territories of Puerto Rico, Guam, and the Virgin Islands). Federal and state governments share responsibility for the new program. Many factors contribute to eligibility, among them being over 65 years of age, legally blind, physically or mentally disabled for work for a period of at least twelve months, for a terminal illness, or for having severely limited income and limited financial resources. Further qualifications demand that recipients live in one of the fifty states or the District of Columbia, and that they are either citizens or aliens who have been lawfully admitted to permanent residence or lawfully admitted in accordance with the Immigration and Nationality Act.

If you believe that your patient may qualify for this assistance, visit the local social security or welfare office for full information and get a copy of the booklet mentioned above. Unless you are unusually sagacious, the booklet alone will be inadequate since the information it gives is sketchy and not a simple matter to interpret. It might be a wise move to send for the pamphlet, read it through, and then be prepared with specific questions when you visit the social security or welfare office.

Medicaid

Eligibility Requirements

A number of states limit Medicaid benefits to those persons who are already living on welfare funds prior to admission to a health-care facility and to those who become eligible for welfare during the course of their institutionalization. Most

states, fortunately, are more liberal and more realistic in awareness of medical need and the potentially disastrous effects on
the financial equilibrium of some individuals and families.
These states offer Medicaid assistance to recipients of supplemental security income (formerly categorized as families with
dependent children, the aged, the blind, and permanently and
totally disabled persons who are medically indigent) and frequently to other needy and low-income people, often including
husbands or wives of qualified persons.

The more liberal states provide Medicaid benefits to persons
who *would be* financially eligible were they not provided with
financial assistance for medical care: in other words, persons
who could continue to meet their routine living expenses independently (in accordance with minimum living standards as
determined by the state) if they were not faced with the additional and sometimes overwhelming burden of medical costs.
Many states will take into account the necessity for an individual or a family to continue to own a home, to drive a car, to
own a modest life insurance policy, or to hold on to a small
financial reserve (an amount under five figures, sometimes
under four). States may, at their own option, grant benefits to
nonresidents.

States differ widely in the range of eligibility requirements
they impose. Generally, however, in addition to financial need,
qualifications for Medicaid assistance in a skilled nursing facility demand that the patient's physician must prescribe the need
for skilled nursing care or observation, the continuous availability of licensed nurses, or other criteria based primarily on
the type of care required rather than the amount. As opposed
to qualifications for Medicare benefits, the patient need not be
hospitalized prior to his admission.

Most states grant Medicaid assistance in skilled nursing facilities to qualified persons 21 years of age or older. A handful of
states provide the exception to the rule by imposing no age
restrictions whatever. These facts apply except for those patients suffering tuberculosis or mental illness.

If there is any possibility that your patient may warrant

Medicaid assistance, then apply directly to the local department of social services or the local welfare office. There you will be given accurate and precise information as to that state's stipulations for enrollment and an itemized list of benefits to which your patient is entitled.

Medicaid Benefits

Adult children are not legally responsible for meeting the costs of their parents' medical care. Legally, financial responsibility is limited to the husband or wife of a patient and to the parents of dependent children under 21 or of older children who are either blind or totally disabled. If you are the patient's brother or sister, his son or daughter or niece or nephew, you may be earning tens of thousands of dollars a year, even hundreds of thousands, yet your patient will still qualify for Medicaid assistance if he personally meets the eligibility requirements of his state.

Further, every Medicaid patient in a nursing home who has no income of his own is granted a minimum personal monthly allowance of at least $25; on occasion up to $33 for recipients of supplemental security income. This sum can be used for such items as dry cleaning, for barber or beautician services, for cigarettes or candy or soda, for expenses incurred during medically authorized visits outside of the nursing home, or any other personal wants.

If your patient is the recipient of social security benefits, or if he has a pension from any source whatever, he will have to contribute all but his monthly allowance to the cost of his nursing-home care. If he has some funds of his own, depending on the state, he may be able to keep $30 a month for his personal use instead of $25. For instance, your patient may have two monthly pension checks: one for $170 from social security and another for $130 from a personal pension, a total of $300 monthly. The monthly bill from the nursing home may be $900. He will then be asked to sign over both his checks to the nursing home. The home is obliged to return $25 (or sometimes $30) to him for spending money and apply the remaining $275 (or $270) against his monthly bill. Medicaid will provide the balance to complete payment to the nursing home. Or perhaps your patient has a bank account of $2,000 or $5,000 or $50,000. In this event he can apply for Medicaid only after he has directly paid the nursing home on a private basis until either such time as his funds are exhausted or, depending on the state's requirements, until they are reduced to an amount that he is permitted to retain and still be eligible for Medicaid benefits.

Incidentally, either the bookkeeping or other specified office should be open to patients at regular and frequent intervals during the week so that a patient can withdraw money from his allowance, cash a check or, perhaps, take his wedding ring from the patients' safe for a weekend at home.

Medicaid-Reimbursed Services

Medicaid covers the full costs of a two- or four-bedded room (or a private room if it is medically prescribed), all meals and snacks including special diet, regular nursing services and sometimes private-duty nursing if it is medically prescribed, recreation, prescribed rehabilitation programs, social services, and other regular programs of the home available under the per diem rate. Coverage extends for as long as the patient qualifies both medically and financially.

Other nursing-home services covered by Medicaid vary in different states but include some or all of the following: physicians' services, podiatry, psychological evaluation and treatment, prescribed drugs, medical equipment, such as wheelchairs, crutches, braces, hearing aids, and prosthetic devices, transportation to and from medical and social services, dental care, optometric care and eyeglasses, laboratory, X-ray, and other diagnostic, screening, and preventive services, and limited chiropractic care.

Medical Review for Medicaid Patients

It is true that regional departments of social service have been depending to a large extent on regularly submitted written reports in order to determine the patient's need for continued stay in a skilled nursing facility. This procedure parallels the evaluation methods used by intermediary organizations in determining patients' needs under the Medicare program. However, Medicaid goes one step further, and it is indeed a giant step in its acknowledgment of the individual and his needs.

In May 1971 Medicaid instituted "Periodic Medical Review and Medical Inspections in Skilled Nursing Homes (and Mental Hospitals)." The review, which is a forerunner of the PSRO program (pages 100-102), is held at least annually and sometimes more frequently. Its purpose is to determine whether or not the patient continues to require the level of care administered in a skilled nursing facility, whether or not he is receiving all the modalities of care that he requires, and whether or not these services meet the highest standards.

The professional team responsible for the annual Medicaid review of patient care is comprised of a physician who heads the group, one or more registered nurses, and a trained social service worker. Further reviews that may be made during the course of the year are sometimes conducted without the physician, in which event the surveyors report back to the director of the program. An integral component of the review team is a behind-the-scenes staff of consultants representing all the professional areas of nursing-home services.

In the effort to view patient conditions as they really are and to observe patient care as it exists on a daily basis, a facility is never notified more than forty-eight hours in advance that such a survey will take place. If serious inadequacies are found, then unannounced inspections may be made at any time.

Members of the review team make personal contact with

every Medicaid patient in the facility, observe his overall grooming and cleanliness and comfort, and converse with him, wherever possible, to assess his attitude and to elicit his evaluation of the services and personnel of the home. Interviews are held with patients and with physicians and other staff members assigned to patient care; and considerable time is devoted to studying the patient's medical records and patient-care plans. If a patient's health status or the quality or extent of his medical care is questioned, the physician of the review team may personally examine the patient and confer with the attending physician, the medical director, or both.

The medical reviews are undertaken by state licensing agencies whereas the PSRO reviews are to be conducted by independent groups and extend to the monitoring of Medicare-reimbursed health care as well as Medicaid. If ample finances and professional manpower are available so that the Professional Standards Review Organizations are enabled to operate on a functional, productive, and frequent basis, substantial gains will have been made over the present inadequate system of medical opinion directing the course of a patient's life on the basis of a few well chosen or ill chosen words. If, however, the PSRO concept does not develop beyond a token basis, its contribution to the long-term patient will be negligible. Surely either the PSRO or the present state-managed medical review must mature into a full-blown meaningful system of accurate control over both Medicare and Medicaid, and one must give way to the other or both will suffer an early demise.

Medicaid: Disallowance of Benefits

Benefits in a skilled nursing facility can be terminated for the Medicaid patient just as they can be terminated for the Medicare patient. This occurs either when it is decided that the patient no longer requires this level of care and that a less costly agency can meet all his needs, or when a patient's financial circumstances take an upward swing. Determination of the patient's nursing and rehabilitation needs is made by the attending physician, the utilization review committee, the local department of social services (based on routine written reports), the medical review team, or the PSRO. Determination of his continued financial need is fixed by state policy.

When a Medicaid patient is disallowed further stay in a nursing home, discharge procedure differs significantly from the Medicare discharge procedure. First, benefits are never discontinued retroactively; second, a "reasonable" amount of time is given for appropriate arrangements to be made for the patient, rather than the three-day cutoff period established by Medicare; third, and perhaps most important, before canceling benefits, Medicaid takes the *whole* person into consideration rather than evaluating his physical status alone. Recognition is given to the patient's social, emotional, and psychological needs, as well as his physical ones. If he is ready to live independently, consideration is given to the time that must be invested to find him a suitable room or apartment or to re-enroll for welfare assistance. If he is to be transferred to an intermediate care facility or to a senior citizens residence, recognition is given to the value of finding suitable placement. If plans are made for him to live with family or friends, a reasonable period is allowed for arrangements to be completed.

Discharge planning plays a prominent role here as it does under all circumstances of determining patients' post-facility needs.

Medicare and Medicaid Together

If your patient is covered by both Medicare and Medicaid, Medicare (Part A) picks up the full tab for the first twenty days of per diem costs in a skilled nursing facility. After the first twenty days, when Medicare imposes a $9 a day deductible to be paid by the patient, in most states Medicaid will pay this co-insurance to recipients of welfare or supplemental security income. At the conclusion of the Medicare benefit period or spell of illness, Medicaid will pick up the full costs for per diem charges and medical services (page 108) for as long as the patient continues to qualify both medically and financially. In every instance where coverage is provided by both programs, Medicare must be billed, must approve the billing, and must submit reimbursement before Medicaid can be approached. The only exception is that the physician may bill Medicaid directly for the $60 annual deductible under Part B of Medicare.

After the patient has received the initial $60 of care covered by Part B, the attending physician must first bill Medicare for 80 percent of his fee, await approval and reimbursement, and then bill Medicaid for up to the remaining 20 percent. (In some states Medicaid allowance is less than 20 percent of the physician's fee.)

The partnership of Medicare and Medicaid in a nursing-home setting can endure for only as long as Medicare approves the patient's stay. At the end of this period Medicare steps out of the picture altogether, and Medicaid has the option of approving or disapproving the patient's further stay and subsequent reimbursement.

Hospital-SNF Contract
Based on Blue Cross

If your patient is to be transferred directly from a hospital to a nursing home, and if he subscribes to Blue Cross, another avenue is open for payment of nursing-home per diem costs. This course is the exception rather than the rule, but it is well worth your inquiry.

Some general hospitals that are members of Blue Cross go into contract with some skilled nursing facilities for nursing-home coverage based on the patient's Blue Cross status. If your patient has a Blue Cross policy covering thirty days of hospital care, for example, and if he has used only ten of them in the hospital, then of course he has twenty days still covered by his policy. Under the hospital-skilled nursing facility contract plan, this policy coverage can be used for twice the remaining number of days in a skilled nursing facility with which the hospital holds such a contract. Thus it is possible, under certain circumstances, that the patient who is eligible for twenty more days of hospital care can replace this benefit with forty days in a nursing home.

In the event that the hospital has such a contract with a nursing home, it is the hospital—not Blue Cross—that would have full information for you and be in a position to inform you of the one or more nursing homes with which it holds such contracts. Benefits of Blue Shield (covering costs of doctors' fees and other professional services not included in the per diem charge) never apply once the patient has left the hospital. Benefits are limited strictly to Blue Cross coverage of daily rates. The hospital's medical social service worker will be in a position to tell you whether or not the hospital holds such a contract and, if it does, with which nursing homes.

Private Payment

If your patient has no pertinent insurance coverage—private, Medicare, Medicaid, or Blue Cross—the only remaining option is direct private payment to the nursing home. One question addressed to the admissions officer or the administrator of the nursing home will bring you an answer as to the daily rate for a private room or for a two-bedded or four-bedded room. Neither federal nor state codes impose any ceilings on these rates for private-paying patients. It is up to your patient and to you to accept the rate or look elsewhere.

The per diem rate *may* be only the beginning. Depending on the individual nursing home, there are many services and supplies that can be charged separately, over and above the daily rate, to a private-paying patient. In a few states these extra charges are governed to a degree, but I strongly urge you to secure a signed list of all extra charges before you admit your patient to any nursing home on a private-paying basis.

In accordance with your patient's needs it may be critical for you to predetermine whether or not there are extra charges for equipment such as a wheelchair, crutches, or a walker; medical and nursing supplies such as oxygen, catheters, gauze pads, enemas, and a host of others; special services such as feeding patients and caring for incontinence.

Many nursing homes include physical, occupational, and speech therapies in their daily rates. Many others do not, and there may be a charge of $10 or $12 or more for a single therapy treatment.

Sometimes nursing homes charge private patients for materials used in occupational therapy or recreation. These should be included in the overall cost of care, but in no event should they be paid for unless the product that the patient makes in either program is one that he chooses to own after its completion.

If your patient requires a special bed or mattress, an individually designed wheelchair, traction or other particular equipment, find out if there is a one-time charge or a monthly charge. If your patient requires a special diet, there should be no extra cost, but don't take it for granted; ask for a commitment.

The fee of the attending physician is a personal matter to be discussed directly with him. But inquire about fees for laboratory and X ray; fees of the nursing home's dentist, podiatrist, and optometrist; possible costs for outside trips that are part and parcel of a recreation program or transportation that may be required for services not available on the premises.

The questions you will want predetermined are so myriad, and cover so broad a spectrum, that the single effective way of establishing full costs is to demand a written signed statement of any and all charges beyond the per diem rate and whether or not these are one-time or repeated charges.

8

Utilization Review

AMONG THE UNPLEASANT DUTIES of a nursing-home administrator are those instances when the closest relative or friend of a patient must be told that the time has come for discharge. Not a preplanned discharge that has been anticipated with pleasure but, rather, one that has come about unexpectedly, precipitously, and without either practical or emotional preparation of the patient or relative. Sometimes the discharge is due to the determination of Medicare or Medicaid review, but more often it is the outcome of a periodic meeting of the utilization review committee.

It's an explosive experience to be told abruptly that you must make other arrangements for a loved one; that you must transfer your brain-damaged son to an intermediate-care facility, your crippled or severely diabetic wife to home-health care, or your aged mother to a senior citizens residence. Just yesterday you thought that your patient's future was secure in the nursing home; today the administrator lets you know how wrong your assumption was. He expresses regret at the sudden turn of events; he offers you professional assistance in making suitable arrangements for your patient; but he states firmly that "the utilization review committee has decided that your patient must leave. He no longer requires skilled nursing care."

The utilization review committee. What is it? Who is it? How can it determine what shall happen to the patient you love? Who has the right to disrupt your plans and your patient's way of life? And why so suddenly?

By answering those questions now, perhaps I can prepare you for such a contingency.

Utilization Review Committee

The process of utilization review is a mandatory condition for federal certification of all skilled nursing facilities. It is a federally regulated mechanism established for two major purposes, both of them for the protection of patients: to restrict and thus reserve the utilization of the facility itself to those patients whose physical health would be endangered by a lesser level of care; and to ensure the appropriate utilization and high professional caliber of component services.

Federal standards call for a minimum of two physicians to comprise the full committee. The medical director or advisory physician can serve as one of these. In an effort to ensure impartial and objective medical consideration of a patient's need for continued care, the law requires that a member physician may have no financial interest in the nursing home and may not conduct the review of his own patient.

The obligations of the committee can be more effectively discharged when there are ex officio members including at least the administrator, the director of nursing, the registered therapists, and the social service worker. These key personnel are equipped to offer constructive discussion and opinion, although only the physicians are empowered to vote. One of the physicians serves as chairman. In my opinion standards should call for at least three physicians rather than two, so that there can always be a majority decision.

The primary duties of the utilization review committee are medical care evaluations and definitions and reviews of extended duration of patient stay. These studies are based on information culled from patients' individual medical records and are designed to make objective determination of whether a patient continues to require skilled nursing care or whether his health has improved or stabilized so that he can be considered for discharge, either to his home or to a less intensive level of care.

Written records of all committee activities are safely filed and maintained and are readily available for inspection by regulatory agencies.

Medical Care Evaluations

The purpose of medical care evaluations, which can be made on an authorized preestablished sample basis, is to ascertain that patients are appropriately admitted, that they are given all the services and care they require for the most effective handling of their infirmities, and that their stays are not prolonged beyond the time necessary for daily skilled nursing and/or professional rehabilitation therapy.

Medical evaluations can extend to other matters of concern to the facility or to the community, such as studying one-leg amputees, for example, to analyze patterns of average lengths of stay for specific age groups, intensity and frequency of therapy programs and rehabilitative nursing, tolerance and adaptability to artificial limbs, patient potential to cope emotionally as well as physically, the role and impact of social service, the scope of discharge planning, etc. At least one study based on patient care within the facility is always a subject of committee research.

Here is a typical medical evaluation of a patient, whose benefits were discontinued by vote of the utilization review committee forty-six days after admission.

Case #7399

84-year-old female admitted 4/26/73 from acute hospital, discharged 6/11/73 after forty-six days.

Admitting Diagnosis: Diabetes Mellitus; Atonic [without tension or tone] Bladder; ASHD [arteriosclerotic heart disease]; Chronic Brain Syndrome.

In addition to the diabetes noted above this patient had a rather severe cystitis [inflammation of the bladder] and chronic congestive heart failure. The attending physician examined the patient at regular monthly intervals, making note of such phenomena as variation in blood pressure, variation in blood sugar, presence of peripheral edema [swelling caused by retention of abnormal amounts of fluid], cardiac status, and status of the bladder infection. At all times during her forty-six-day stay at this facility, the patient was under a considerable volume of medicinal, medical, and skilled nursing care because of her continuing acute and chronic medical signs and symptoms.

The patient was given instruction by R.N.s in independent insulin injection which she was able to master in approximately four weeks. She and her daughter were given detailed dietary instruction and full instructions and information relative to her insulin and other daily medications.

She had been almost altogether confined to bed during her prior five-week stay in the general hospital and was in a severely weakened condition upon admission. Physical therapy for improvement in ambulation was prescribed and administered five mornings a week for fifteen-minute sessions and supported by restorative nursing in daily practice sessions each afternoon.

On 5/14 the patient was referred to the optometrist who found the need for a stronger prescription for reading glasses. These were made for her and fitted on 5/23.

She was referred to the podiatrist on 5/4 and 5/11 for

detailed instruction in foot hygiene. He pared one corn on the right great toe.

On 6/11 she was discharged to her daughter's home; the diabetic and cardiac conditions under control, and the bladder infection cured.

A review of this type is conducted periodically for every Medicare and Medicaid patient. The patterns of care that emerge from such summaries offer valuable potential for analysis of facility services and for the appropriateness and effectiveness of their usage for different infirmities and age groups.

Duration of Stay

Review of duration of stay is the function of the committee that is most apt to directly affect your patient. Every Medicare and Medicaid patient is periodically reviewed by the committee to determine whether or not further stay in the facility is medically indicated. Government compensation to the nursing home is dependent on documented proof of the patient's medical need. According to federal law this review is not mandated for private-paying patients, since public funds are not at stake. Nevertheless, I would like to see such review required for all patients so that the maximum number of beds would always be available to those with genuine medical need, and so that private-paying would not be unnecessarily confined.

When the facility's utilization review plan is first drawn up and submitted to the licensing agency for approval, extended duration of stay is specifically defined in terms of numbers of days. It may be that the same number will be used to cover extended duration for all patients; or it may be that different numbers of days will apply to patients consistent with categories of illness or handicap. According to federal regulations, almost every Medicaid patient is first reviewed by the committee within twenty-one days after admission, and subsequently at intervals of at least thirty days during the first three months, and at intervals of at least ninety days after the first three months. Medicare patients are usually reviewed at more frequent intervals.

Committee Decision to Terminate Duration of Stay

Committee determination that a patient no longer requires the level of care provided by the skilled nursing facility must be the joint decision of two member physicians. Regulations require that one or both of these doctors must consult with the patient's attending physician. Consideration is given to the attending physician's evaluation of the patient's needs, and substantial documentation is required to overrule his opinion. Within forty-eight hours of the committee's decision, written notification of discharge must be submitted to the administrator, the attending physician, and to the patient and/or his closest relative or friend. Final decision as to the disposition of the case must be made no later than seven days after the committee has decided to discontinue benefits. The effect of such determination varies with Medicare and Medicaid beneficiaries, as discussed in Chapter 7.

Full focus is now centered on the discharge plan and the sociomedical summary that have been continuously updated during the course of the patient's stay. Time for action is short, but the goal has been set, and the destination is in sight.

The utilization review committee meets at least monthly and has access to all patients' medical records, patient-care plans, and discharge plans. Discussion centered around any one patient is obviously facilitated and amplified when the physical therapist, for instance, is a member of the group and can add his comments concerning the patient's state of progress, or when the nursing director is there to cite specific instances of improvement or deterioration in the patient's health status.

It is almost invariably a necessity to hold interim utilization reviews. Change in.a patient's condition can occur a week after his case is subject to review or six weeks before he is due for re-evaluation. In these instances two committee physicians must conduct an interim review and report their findings to the administrator. If they determine that the patient is to be discharged from the facility, or that his Medicare or Medicaid benefits will no longer cover his care, then the same rules of notification apply as when this decision is made at a monthly committee meeting. Review of a patient's case must be conducted no later than seven days after the date established by the utilization review plan.

Reviews determining length of stay are also conducted by the committee when an attending physician has decided and documented that he need visit his patient only once every two months (page 54). Then the patient's need for skilled nursing or rehabilitation therapy must be reexamined, and the possibility of his discharge to an intermediate care or other facility must be considered.

Utilization Review Conducted Outside the Facility

Frequently an outside resource, approved by the licensing agency, takes over the process of the facility's utilization review. I not only endorse this policy but would like to see a mandatory requirement that the utilization review committee be composed of *three* physicians from an *outside* resource (local medical society, hospital, or other) who would be supplied with all necessary patient records and supported through the actual presence and participation of the facility's key professional personnel involved with the patient's care.

The combination of physicians from outside the facility and ex officio committee members from within the facility should safeguard the patients' interests. Professionals serving on the staff of the nursing home are equipped to know and understand the patients' physical and emotional health problems and in a position to fully inform the physicians on any and all factors evoking their concern. The physicians, as the decision makers, are better able to remain impartial since they are unfamiliar with the patients themselves or even with the patients' names.

It is a federal requirement that a patient's review be conducted by number or other designation but without referral to that patient's name. However, the committee seldom operates in this manner. Somewhere in the course of discussion, a committee participant will ask, "Is that Mrs. F. that you're talking about? Because if it is, she has a special problem. . . ." Or the social service worker may say, "I think you're probably referring to Mr. R. I agree that he's ready for discharge home, but his wife is in the hospital now, and we can't send him home alone with nobody to care for him. We'll have to make other arrangements."

The use of the patient's name is actually of great value since most people sitting around the table know Mrs. F. or Mr. R. but are not familiar with #7213 or #7485. Patient identity allows for broader, more pertinent, and more accurate discussion and decision since personal knowledge of the patient infallibly brings to the minds of committee members one or more facts not necessarily included in the written records or facts viewed quite differently by various members of the committee.

However, there is a drawback to this procedure that leads me to believe that final decision-making must be in the hands of physicians who are not on the staff of the nursing home and therefore not subject (or considerably less likely to be subject) to the nursing home's influence.

It is an unfortunate but not uncommon occurrence that an administrator or occasionally another committee participant is instructed by an owner to point discussion of a particular case toward a predetermined conclusion. For instance, "Don't let Mrs. L. get away from us. She's so easy to take care of, no trouble to anyone. Dr. X. will help you if you talk to him first. But whatever you do, don't let her go. We need more patients like her."

Or consider the experience of a nursing-home administrator who is a 32-year-old woman, attractive, and unmarried. She confided that it was awfully hard to hold on to Mr. A.; he really didn't need further nursing or rehabilitation care but, she added, "His friend from the city comes up two and three times a week to visit him, and he's great! He takes me out for cocktails and dinner every time, and I'm not about to give that up!"

Selfish motivation frequently affects committee action when physicians and ex officio members are all on the staff of the facility and are familiar with the patient and his family and with each other. This sort of manipulation, which requires the cooperation of the committee physicians, destroys the purpose and the essence of utilization review and wastes governmental funds and taxpayers' monies. Most important of all, it is unjust to those patients who need the professional care offered by the skilled nursing facility but are denied admission because beds are occupied by patients who should be discharged; and it is equally unjust to those patients who should be promoted to a lesser level of care and an increased opportunity to develop independence. Physicians and thus committee chairmanship from an outside source would automatically censor such procedure since this is "dirty linen" not exposed to outsiders. At the same time, committee representation by staff members of the facility would provide recognition of the patients' personal strengths and weaknesses, both physical and emotional.

In some instances, then, you may well be concerned that your patient is being confined beyond the time required by his illness or handicap. But the reverse is not true. He will not be discharged any sooner than necessary unless he happens to be a private-paying patient who presents constant and insoluble problems for the staff. A Medicare or Medicaid patient will not be accepted by an intermediate-care facility or other lesser-care agency if he still requires daily skilled nursing or rehabilitation therapy. If your patient is private paying, he is billed a per diem rate higher than the one established for Medicare or

Medicaid patients, and the facility will be eager to hold on to him unless the situation is untenable.

It is to be hoped that the scope and frequency of the Medical Review established by Professional Standards Review Organizations (pages 100–102) will be developed to fully supplement the utilization review procedure and serve as a regulatory device in assuring its intended purpose.

Discharge Planning

Discharge planning fits hand in glove with the goals of utilization review. An idealistic and thoroughly honest use of the two mechanisms would serve to provide the maximum number of patients with the highest level of care warranted at the lowest possible cost to government and taxpayers.

Discharge planning has always been a responsibility of the conscientiously operated skilled nursing facility: not solely a question of when (or if) to discharge a patient, but professional planning toward the most advantageous placement for the patient once he leaves the facility. The physical health and emotional stamina of the patient are perhaps the most important contributory components, but integral to the total picture are the questions of whether or not he has family members to help care for him, whether he lives in a room located up two flights of stairs, whether he will continue to require therapy treatments for a lower or upper extremity, whether or not he has achieved a meaningful level of independence in the activities of daily living, and other similar factors.

The attending physician, in projecting his long-term goals for the patient, plans ahead toward the most effectual placement for him after discharge from the nursing home. As time goes by, the discharge plan is modified in accordance with the course of the patient's physical and mental progress or deterioration as evaluated by the attending physician, licensed nurses, therapists, social service worker, and any other professionals whose treatment and subsequent entries in the patient's medical record are pertinent to his post-facility placement.

The Department of Health, Education and Welfare has now imposed specific regulations to govern discharge planning designed to meet the patient's individual post-discharge needs. The attending physician must inaugurate the plan within seven days of the patient's admission; the utilization review committee must, at predetermined time intervals, conduct periodic reviews of all discharge plans as well as the procedures established by the facility for effecting and maintaining them. Operational responsibility is specifically assigned to individual staff members or to an outside agency (health, social, or welfare), and appropriate local resources are contacted for assistance in developing and implementing the plans.

At the time of the patient's discharge, the facility provides to the agency or persons responsible for the patient's continued care all current information relative to diagnoses, prior treatment, rehabilitation potential, physician advice concerning immediate care, and pertinent social information.

Patient-Care Policies Committee

In addition to the utilization review committee, federal regulations require certain other standing committees. The only one that will be of direct interest to you is the Patient Care Policies Committee. This committee develops and periodically reviews and modifies patient care policies designed to meet the patients' total needs. Federal regulations call for committee membership to include one or more physicians and one or more registered nurses. It is my opinion that in order to achieve the goal of providing for patients' total needs, committee membership should include administration and all areas of patient care such as rehabilitation services, dietary, recreation, and social services, as well as medical and nursing.

This committee is charged with reviewing policies developed by the medical director or organized medical staff to govern medical, nursing, and other services; and with establishing facility policies for patient admission, transfer, and discharge; for range of services; for frequency of physician visits according to category of patients; and for protection of patients' personal and property rights.

Although federal regulations point to only this general coverage, an effective patient care policies committee will concern itself with a broad spectrum of policies to include medical, nursing, dietary, rehabilitative, pharmaceutical, and diagnostic services. It will supplement the efforts of the infections control committee by establishing procedures for all emergencies, and for critically (not necessarily contagiously) ill or mentally disturbed patients. The committee will also address itself to policies of dental, podiatric, and optometric care, social services, recreation, medical records, transfer agreements, and utilization review.

Federal regulations demand that the committee meets at least annually to review and update policies, but effectiveness of total care for the total patient would indicate a necessity for more frequent meetings. Minutes of all meetings are safely maintained and made available for inspection by regulatory agencies.

Responsibility for the execution of established patient care policies is relegated to one or more physicians or to a registered nurse working under the guidance of an advisory physician.

These written patient care policies are available to the public, as well as to admitting physicians, sponsoring agencies, and patients. I strongly urge you to ask to read a copy of these written policies, bear them in mind, and question any acts or any attitudes that indicate they are being overlooked or overridden by the administration or members of the staff.

Other standing committees required by federal law are Infection Control and Pharmaceutical Services.

9

Admission Day: Before, During, and After

I HAD JUST COME DOWNSTAIRS from making rounds one winter afternoon when the admissions clerk called out to me, "Please come in. Maybe you can help."

I walked into the office. There, strapped in her wheelchair, sat Mrs. Kirk, the patient whom we had been planning to admit. Mrs. Kirk was a woman in her mid-70s. Her plump figure was wedged into the chair by the thick brown fur of her coat. At the moment that I walked through the door Mrs. Kirk was straining her head forward at the neck, her cheeks and her eyes were brightened by her rage, her arms were flailing the air as though they were independent agents, and she was sputtering sounds of frustrated indignation.

Mrs. Kirk had suffered from progressive rheumatoid arthritis most of her adult life. She had been widowed almost a dozen years earlier, and since then she had lived with her daughter and her daughter's husband and their three children. Her daughter was with her now—Ellen Daisley, a woman of about 40, trim, well groomed, and at the moment, troubled and a little teary. She was addressing her words to her mother, but she kept glancing at the admissions clerk and at me, as though for approval of how she was managing.

"Mamma, I know I said I was just taking you for a ride, but what else could I *do?* You never would have come if I'd told you I was taking you to a nursing home."

Mrs. Kirk sobbed convulsively.

A young nurse's aide entered the room and took the suitcase offered her by Mrs. Daisley.

"Mamma, the aide will take your suitcase for you. Yes, I packed it last night after you were asleep. If you want anything more from home, I'll bring it with me tomorrow. You go ahead now, and I'll be there with you in a few minutes."

The aide accompanied the weeping Mrs. Kirk out of the admissions office toward the elevator and the two-bedded room upstairs.

Mrs. Kirk's daughter turned directly to me. "You understand, don't you?" she queried. "Mamma's been living with us for over eleven years now, and it's gotten too much for all of us. Joe and I can never get away for vacations or even weekends anymore, and we worry even when we just go out to dinner. And the children are all busy with their own lives. Anyhow, her arthritis is so much worse than it ever was before. She's really crippled now; she can't do anything for herself, and if I keep trying to take care of her I'll go to pieces altogether, and what will happen to Joe and the children? Even the doctor said she should go to a nursing home."

"Why didn't you tell her the truth?" I asked.

"The truth?" Mrs. Daisley's face mirrored her horror. "Oh, I couldn't hurt her feelings like *that,*" she gasped. "After all, she's my mother."

Sound farfetched? It isn't. There are many Mrs. Daisleys who don't know how to tell their mothers or fathers or husbands that nursing care and a nursing home have become necessities. They know that the pronouncement will bring with it a sense of rejection. All the powers of reason, the need of the family to return to an independent unit, the doctor's instructions, and, most of all, the physical debility of their loved ones point to a nursing home as the only logical solution to a web of problems. But logic has never been a handmaiden to emotion, and the many Mrs. Daisleys are so ridden with guilt at not continuing to "take care of Mamma" that they run from facing the facts and veritably dump their loved ones at the door of the nursing home with a prayer that somehow things will "work out." The trauma and the feeling of rejection that "Mamma" will experience is multiplied a thousandfold because now she *has* been rejected: rejected as a human being with the right to know and understand where she is going to live and why; the right to partake in the thought and planning and decision-making; the right to evidence her maturity and even self-sacrifice, if you will, out of her years of life-wisdom and her love for her family.

Now it's another day and another new patient. This time I find a Mrs. Morris sitting in a wheelchair waiting to be admitted. She is in her early 70s, and her husband is with her, talking to the admissions officer. Mrs. Morris has arrived directly from the hospital. She is sitting quietly, her face expressionless.

As with Mrs. Kirk, Mrs. Morris has suffered rheumatoid arthritis for many years, and its crippling effects have become progressively more severe. Although almost her total body has been afflicted, the intense pain and the uselessness of her hands had become unbearable to her. Finally her physician recommended surgery in the hope of restoring some use to the fingers of her right hands. The effects of the surgery were painful, incredibly slow to heal, and totally unsuccessful. Mrs. Morris' hand remained as useless as it had been before the operation and temporarily even more painful. The surgeon put her on chemotherapy, with heavy dosages of cortisone to which Mrs. Morris had a severe reaction. The combination of pain, pain-killers, allergic response to medications, and many weeks of confinement to bed all added to her general debility and apparently hastened the deterioration of her bladder muscles. Now

Mrs. Morris was incontinent of urine, and there was little hope that this condition would ever reverse itself.

She was sicker and weaker than she had been at any time in her life. She was depressed, unmotivated, and utterly indifferent when her doctor told her that she would have to be transferred to a nursing home. He told Mrs. Morris just the day before the transfer was to be made. He made no mention of how long she might have to stay, and Mrs. Morris asked no questions because she had no interest. The doctor had told her husband only two or three days earlier, but he had forewarned Mr. Morris that his wife might well spend the rest of her life as a nursing-home patient. She might live for a good number of years—her condition in no way threatened her life—but he felt that further deterioration was inevitable, and that she would progressively need increased nursing care during the course of time.

The news came as a heavy blow to Mr. Morris. How to accept this affront to a way of life—his wife confined to a nursing home for the rest of her days? Mr. Morris struggled to accept the fact, but what he was able to accept logically, he could not accept emotionally. So on the day of admission to the nursing home Mr. Morris said to his wife, "Don't worry, darling. You'll only be here for a week or two, and then you'll come back home with me." How could he possibly hurt his beloved wife by allowing her to feel that he would leave her at the nursing home for more than a short stay?

But the week or two would pass. Inevitably there would be questions: "Am I going home soon now? When will I be getting better? When will I leave here?" Mr. Morris would have the option of breaking the news then, and admitting that he had misrepresented the facts, or continuing the lie of "just a few weeks more."

Before Admission Day

The circumstances of putting a loved one into a nursing home vary with every admission. You may have weeks to prepare your patient, or you may have only a day or two. Your patient may be slated for a stay of a few weeks, or he may have to be institutionalized for months or years or the remainder of his lifetime. Your patient may be lucid and intelligent and questioning, or he may be utterly apathetic or confused or brain-damaged. He may be in his 60s or in his 80s; on the other hand he may be 22.

The details of what you tell your patient, when you tell him, and how you do it are up to you and are surely governed in large part by his emotional stamina and the kind of relationship you have with him. There is only one piece of advice I can give you with absolute certainty: whatever you do, whatever you say, be honest with him. Before you can be honest with him, you must be honest with yourself; before you can prepare him, you must prepare yourself.

Honesty should be and of course actually is an absolute. Being a little bit honest is like being a little bit pregnant. But certainly there will be times when, in the best interest of your patient, it may be necessary to tell only a part of the truth, a part of the story. As much as you tell him, stick to the truth as a basic. You know your patient best. It may be easier for him in the long run if you tell him right away that there is little or no hope of his ever being discharged from the nursing home, "and so we will work together to try to make it a comfortable experience for you. I'll help in every way I can." For many patients this could be too difficult a burden to handle. Then honesty might best be diluted by saying, "We really don't know yet how long you'll have to stay. Let's just take it a week or so at a time, and not look too far ahead." The urgent necessity here is to avoid the outright lie and the offer of an unfeasible hope that "it will be only a few weeks."

This principle applies whether your patient is young or old, lucid or confused. Earlier in the text I stressed the importance for the nursing-home staff to treat patients as human beings, affording them the dignity and respect of individuals with inalienable rights of their own. Certainly this is your responsibility, too. Don't belittle your patient, don't treat him as a whining, wheedling infant who must be assured right here and now that he will have his own way. If he has any maturity at all, even if he is still young, he has learned that he doesn't and can't always have things his way. Don't let him embark on this difficult and lonely and unnatural journey with the added impediment of false hope. On the contrary, fortify him with your respect for his strengths (as well as your understanding and acceptance of his weaknesses), your awareness of his ego and his ego needs, and your continuance of the relationship you shared with him before he became ill. Let him know now, and again and again, that he remains the same *person* to you that he always was and that *you* need to continue the same relationship with him that you've had in the past.

Afford him this same courtesy and respect if he is disoriented or aphasic. It is truly impossible for you or anyone else to estimate the exact extent of his awareness. But even if your words are gibberish to him, he will know your attitude, sense your feelings of closeness or withdrawal, and rely heavily on your love and acceptance of him as he is now.

If time allows—as it probably will if you're admitting your patient directly from home—and if his physical and mental conditions permit, bring him to the nursing home well before the day of admission and take him on a full tour. If for any reason the nursing home objects to your doing this, then you object to the nursing home and forget that particular facility altogether.

It won't be practical to bring your patient with you on your initial shopping expedition while you are evaluating various homes. But if you narrow down your choice to two or three, urge him to come with you to make the final determination for himself. If his illness or disability prohibits this possibility, then talk with him about the investigation you have made and discuss those facilities that interest you. It may be that ABC Manor offers more than any of the other homes you've visited. It has the most cheerful atmosphere, the most tempting menus, the best staffed nursing department, and the widest variety of programs, but it's located at a distance where you will have to limit visiting to two or three times or maybe just once a week. On the other hand, the XYZ Nursing Home offers adequate although not outstanding services, but it's located in the immediate neighborhood and you can come by every day. Describe the two to him in detail, the advantages and disadvantages of each, and let him make the choice for himself. Be sure to tell him that his selection need not be permanent; you can always make arrangements to transfer him elsewhere. If his physician sends him to a nursing home directly from the hospital, with no time for you to shop beforehand, let him know that the doctor's selection need not be final.

Encourage him to talk as much as he wants of his fears and doubts. Listen attentively and really hear what he says. Don't belittle his intelligence by assurances that everything will be just fine and he has no reason to worry. He has ample reason to worry, and both of you know it. Evidence your respect for him as the person he always has been by appreciating his fears and letting him realize that you do. You may have to say, "Yes, I've wondered about that, too. Let's hope it will work out, but even if it doesn't, you know that I'll help you in any way I can." If you attempt to swoosh away his fears with a homily or a cliché, you deny him his status as an individual in his own right.

If your patient is disoriented or aphasic to the point where there is no basis for any kind of communication, you will have to do the thinking for him. But talk to him, tell him why and how the decisions were made, discuss with him both the nursing home that has been selected and the reasons for his projected stay. He *may* understand some of what you're saying; he *will* sense that you're holding a discussion with him on a level of equality. And by all means, take him with you to see the nursing home before he is admitted (unless he is sent directly from the hospital) so that there is the possibility of an aura of familiarity on the day of his admission.

Day of Admission

The day of admission will be a difficult one for your patient (and for you, too). There is no way to make it easy for him, but there are ways to make it a little less difficult. Most important, be *with* him. If he's coming directly from home, it's an easy matter for you to take him, even if it means using an ambulance or asking another person to come along to help. If he's being sent directly from a hospital, ride along with him in the ambulance if you're permitted. Otherwise, be waiting for him at the nursing home when he arrives.

Either you or he will be required to spend some time with the admissions officer, answering questions that are necessary to complete the admissions form. It may be that your patient's physical condition will necessitate his being brought to his room and put directly to bed. If that is not the case, let him stay with you. If he is disoriented or aphasic, he will at least be at your side and not wondering what it is that you're doing, or what it is that he's doing alone and in a strange place. If he is lucid, let him answer the questions that are asked. Always, under all circumstances, let him do as much of anything and everything as he is capable of doing for himself. Keep uppermost in your mind the grave importance of helping him to feel useful and of value to himself and to others.

Go with him to his room. We cannot imagine any nursing

home that would disallow this because of visiting hour restrictions. This is a point you might want to raise with nursing-home personnel before admission day. Any home that would prohibit you from being with your patient from the moment of admission until at least the close of visiting hours is a nursing home that cannot possibly recognize the human needs of its patients, and it does not warrant your trust.

A reputable nursing home will make every effort to place patients with congenial roommates. However, this may not be possible on the first day; there may be only one bed available. Most nursing homes have one-bedded (private), two-bedded, and four-bedded rooms. You may have to compromise with other than your choice until a bed is available where you want it. So your patient may be happy with the room he is given, or he may not be. It's highly probable that on this first day he won't be too happy with any arrangements or with any roommate. For the moment, this must be secondary.

A number of nursing homes have welcoming committees comprised of patients who come by to greet a new patient and later, sometimes the same day but more probably the next, introduce him to other patients and show him around the home.

Whether or not such a committee exists, you can be helpful to your patient in this regard, if not on the day of admission, then soon after. But on this first day, there will undoubtedly be times when you will be away from him. The physician may want to examine him, there may be tests to be performed, or other reasons why you will be asked to step out of his room for a while. Or he may want to take a nap. Use this time to go into the dayroom and socialize with some of the patients on his nursing floor. If you're lucky, you can boost his morale beautifully by being able to report that you talked with a Mr. Zilch who has a room just down the hall, and that Mr. Zilch is also a mechanical engineer or also a drygoods salesman or construction worker or whatever; that he and your patient should have a lot in common, and that perhaps they'll meet each other tomorrow. Or perhaps you'll meet a patient with the same hobby, the same set of family circumstances, or the same background of illness or disability.

Stay with your patient all that day, until the last possible moment. Leave his room when necessary; come back to it as soon as you can. Unpack his clothes for him, and ask him where he wants you to put his robe and slippers, or his pajamas or toilet articles. Ask if he's thought of something else he might want you to bring from home tomorrow; or is there something you can bring him now from the canteen or a local store.

Incidentally, there will be regulations affecting what you may or may not bring him by way of food, and chances are that whatever you bring you will have to leave at the nursing station, marked with his name, for members of the nursing staff to give to him at appropriate times. Inquire about the details from the charge nurse and tell your patient what the rules are; what you may or may not bring to him and what he must do to get the crackers or fruit after you do bring them in.

Don't bring too many clothes or other items on the day of admission. Storage space will be minimal, and it will be a nuisance to him—and to the staff—if you overload him with more than he needs. You can always bring more as time goes by. Supply him with enough changes for a week. Personal laundry will be done for him at the home, probably at least twice a week, so he won't need too much. Items of clothing should all be drip-dry since it is doubtful that many homes do any ironing these days. Every item of clothing should be clearly marked with his name, using indelible ink rather than sewed on tape that can loosen and come off in the wash. Prepare two lists of all his belongings and describe each item briefly. In other words "one sweater" is not sufficiently descriptive. Far better to write "one gray wool V-neck cardigan." Include items such as upper or lower dentures, eyeglasses, hearing aid, etc. Give one of these lists to the charge nurse and the other to your patient. It's a good idea to have staff members aware that he knows—and you know—exactly what possessions he has with him; and the list can prove valuable if any items are lost.

Such a list will in no way prevent petty thievery and, unfortunately, a great deal of this goes on in hospitals and in nursing homes. There isn't a thing you can do personally to prevent it. You can only guard against the effect of its impact by seeing to it that the wristwatch he wears is an inexpensive one, that all the items he brings with him are replaceable at moderate cost, and that nothing is actually *ir*replaceable. The only cash he will need is for the possible purchase of small items at the canteen. The nursing home is *not* responsible for loss or theft.

According to the furnishings in his room, and the amount of tabletop space, he may want a photograph of you or his children or of other persons he holds dear. There may be a knick-knack of some sort that has special meaning to him, and that you can bring with you another day. Let him settle in his room, though, before you bring anything beyond the essentials; let him determine for himself if he prefers uncluttered space for his book and eyeglasses or pen and paper or if he would rather have that picture or the little statuette he has always cherished.

If you can arrange to have some privacy with him—and by all means, try—encourage him to talk before you leave. It may well be that he has nothing he wants to say on this first day, or he may have such a host of conflicting thoughts and emotions that he's not ready to sort them out and discuss them with you. Don't press him. But make sure that you give him the opportunity to talk, that you let him know you're interested in his first reactions and want to share them with him. And again, listen and hear and understand and respect.

After Admission

"After admission" can be a long, long time. If it's only a matter of a few weeks, there is really no problem. If, however, his stay is to be for many months or many years, your work is cut out for you.

Your primary responsibility is to maintain with him the same kind of a relationship you had before he was institutionalized. The same *kind* of relationship. It can't be exactly what it used to be, because circumstances have changed in a drastic manner, but keep it as close to what it was as is humanly possible.

A basic fundamental toward accomplishing this is a long and thorough discussion with your patient's attending physician. The more you can fully understand the effects of his illness, the easier it will be for you to relate to him. If you can understand, for instance, that the newly developed and highly volatile temper your patient displays is due to a bodily misfunction or attendant brain damage, then you need not feel guilty or defensive when he raises his voice or verbally attacks you. The more accepting you can be, the more quickly such a mood will pass. If you feel threatened by his temper, frustrated or rejected, then your reactions will serve to irritate and exaggerate his, and you will have created an emotional seesaw that could be avoided—or, at least, minimized—by understanding and stability on your part.

If your patient is senile or aphasic, both of you will suffer heartbreaking frustration. The more information and the more understanding that your doctor will give you by explaining the facts, the better able you will be to maintain a stable and still meaningful relationship.

You may want to call on the help of the home's social service worker who will be in a position to explain your patient's psychological reactions and your own. Don't hesitate to ask for this assistance. It's not a sign of weakness on your part, but, rather, a sign of strength in your determination to make the nursing-home experience a successful one.

If the patient is your husband, and he's a devoted father to your two teen-agers, bring the children with you as often as you can or have them visit on the days when you can't get there.

Talk to him about the children and ask his advice in those matters where you have been accustomed to seeking his opinion. Don't make the mistake of trying to shield him from all the problems. He will feel left out, unimportant, unwanted. Help him to continue in the role he played before he became ill. It's not only fair to ask him, "What should I do about Johnny? He'll never make college next fall unless he starts to apply himself to his schoolwork"; it's unfair to your husband if you don't consult with him. He is still the same person he was; he is still concerned with his son, and he is still in need of retaining his status in the family. If Johnny has 104-degree temperature, and the doctor doesn't know what's causing it, then certainly you needn't burden your husband with the worry, but here again is a time for "diluted honesty" when you can tell him that Johnny is in bed with a slight fever, and you're hoping he'll be fine in a few days. On the other hand, if it happens that your husband has been a practicing physician, then he deserves the full truth so that he can have the opportunity to live his rightful role.

If he's accustomed to handling the checkbook and paying all the bills then, unless his illness is so severe as to prohibit the possibility, ask him if he would please *help you* by continuing to take care of the finances. Reaffirm your faith in him as the person he has always been and so let him reaffirm his faith in himself.

If your patient is your mother and has always devoted herself to housekeeping, cooking, and shopping, ask her how you can prepare goulash the way she always did, yours never turns out to be as good as hers; or what furniture polish she found the best; or is $1.65 too much to pay for a box of whatever. If your patient is a son or daughter, or a close friend, talk about a hobby or special interest and ask questions, ask advice. Bring in clippings from magazines or newspapers and start off a conversation with "You know more about this than I. Do you agree with this article? Why?"

I look back to a time in my own life when I wasn't ill or in-

stitutionalized, but when I was in the midst of deep and serious personal difficulty. My friends all sought to protect me by
not "adding" their burdens to mine. The attitude was "She
has enough on her shoulders, I won't tell her about my problems." They were so wrong. I clearly recall that through those
years I felt that I was the only one who had trouble. All my
close friends who had always confided in me in the past appeared suddenly to have no problems at all. I felt that their
lives were running smoothly in every aspect, while mine was
running smoothly in none. How much better off I would have
been, how much more easily I could have coped with my own
affairs if they had continued to let me share their lives with
them and allowed me to continue to give of myself. In their efforts to spare me, they put me in an unfamiliar role where I
felt shut off and alone.

In the same vein, it's a misguided kindness to "take over" for
a patient. I remember a Mr. Oliver who came to our nursing
home after major hip surgery. He was in his late 30s, a successful junior partner in a law firm. He was good humored, alert,
interested in the people around him and in the political affairs
of the world. His wife was attractive and bright and charming.
She was a high school teacher and came to visit him every
evening.

In an honest effort to make life easier for him, to try to com-
pensate for what he was missing in the world outside, she did
everything *for* him that she could. She fussed over smoothing
his bedclothes and straightening his drawers. She insisted on
answering his mail to spare him the "trouble." She interceded
on his behalf with doctor, nurse, therapist, and aides. And she
went out of her way to spare him any discussions of the small
everyday problems relating to her work where she had formerly
always sought his advice. She chatted to him about nothings;
she responded to his doubts and complaints with "Oh, that's
not so bad; it will soon be over." She urged him not to worry
about what might be going on in his office and not to excite
himself with political events. She confined their conversations

together to what he had eaten for lunch, did he need new pajamas, was the night nurse being more pleasant, and could she plump his pillow to make him more comfortable.

Slowly and steadily she made him dependent, listless, unmotivated. His loss of ego strength brought about a general deterioration. He became uncooperative in his physical therapy sessions, uninterested in joining recreation programs or participating in social activities; he became consistently more apathetic and willing to lie in bed as long as the nurses would permit him.

Mrs. Oliver had emasculated her husband by depriving him of all decision-making, all advisory discussion, all responsibility. She could have been instrumental in strengthening his motivation and thus his recovery had she fortified his role as husband and man and offered him the opportunity to continue to give of himself despite his role as patient.

Feelings of guilt often lead relatives to respond in the same manner as Mrs. Oliver. They take away all patient responsibility and ego along with it, and they antagonize the staff in their demanding attitudes that are nothing more than escape hatches for their own guilt.

During the first week or so of your patient's stay he will probably want you to do for him, until he has made at least an initial adjustment. But stop taking over for him at the earliest possible moment. The one real gift you can make to him is allowing him to give of himself, and that is possible only if you allow him to retain his old role and his sense of self-worth. Of course, if you have been the dominant one all along, if he has always looked to you for guidance, decision-making and "ruling the roost," then your obligation is to maintain his confidence by continuing to play the role that initially made him comfortable.

Continue to live your own life as fully as you can. You'll be a more interesting person when you come to visit. You'll have news to report, questions to ask, anecdotes to tell. Being busy and interested and productive can have a contagious effect and, almost without doubt, your patient will respond by being busier and more interested and more productive within the confines of the nursing home and the limitations of his disability.

Urge his friends to visit as often as they can and to send frequent cards or notes. There's nothing wrong with a little bribery if you ask a friend of his to "come over for dinner, and then we'll go together to the nursing home." Or call a friend to ask him to please visit on Sunday if there's a reason you can't get over that day.

Don't expect your patient to be enthusiastic about his stay in the nursing home. If he is, that's pure gravy, and say a humble prayer of thanks. It's more practical to think in terms of helping him adjust by explaining the reasons for some of the problems or by discussing with him what alternatives there may be in coping with them.

Your job is to help him to be as contented as is reasonably possible, to provide motivation for recovery and for life itself through keeping him consciously aware of your respect and your need for him, and reinforcing his faith in himself as a valuable human being.

10

Patients' Bill of Rights

IN 1973 the American Hospital Association issued a bill of rights for hospital patients. A year later the Department of Health, Education and Welfare announced enforcement of an equivalent bill itemizing rights and responsibilities of long-term patients. As a new requirement for federal licensure of skilled nursing facilities, copies are to be available to all patients, to their responsible relatives, friends, sponsoring agencies, and representative payees, and to the public. To the owners or trustees of the nursing facility is delegated the responsibility for establishing pertinent written policies, and to the administrator is delegated the responsibility for developing and adhering to applicable procedures and for ensuring that "the staff of the facility be trained and involved in the implementation of these policies and procedures."

In presenting these rights I will attempt to modify some of the rhetorical language. However, the frequent use of quotation marks indicates exact quotation from the Federal Register of October 3, 1974 (Vol. 39, No. 193, Part II) issued by the Department of Health, Education and Welfare relative to skilled nursing facilities.

Itemized Rights

Fourteen specific rights are mandated. The first four of these are delegated also to the patient's "guardian, next of kin, sponsoring agency(ies) or representative payee (except when the facility itself is representative payee)" particularly in the event that the patient is disoriented, aphasic, or otherwise judged by his attending physician to be incompetent or "medically incapable of understanding these rights."

In accordance with federal regulations, effective as of December 2, 1974, every patient in a skilled nursing facility shall have the right:

1. To know and understand "as evidenced by [his] written acknowledgement" all his rights and responsibilities as a patient, and all "rules and regulations governing patient conduct and responsibilities" either before or at the time of his admission and during the course of his stay;

2. To be fully informed, either before or on the day of his admission, and during the course of his stay, of all services offered by the facility, and of all charges not covered by Medicare or Medicaid, or by the basic per diem rate;

3. To be kept "fully informed, by a physician, of his medical condition unless medically contraindicated (as documented by a physician, in his medical record), and [be] afforded the opportunity to participate in the planning of his medical treatment and to refuse to participate in experimental research";

4. To be given "reasonable advance notice" of any transfer or discharge from the facility, and the right to be secure in the knowledge that such transfer or discharge will be made "only for medical reasons, or for his welfare or that

of other patients, or for nonpayment for his stay" except where prohibited by Medicare or Medicaid, and that "all such actions [be] documented in his medical record";

5. To be "encouraged and assisted, throughout his period of stay, to exercise his rights as a patient and as a citizen and to this end [be granted the right to] voice grievances and recommend changes in policies and services to facility staff and/or outside representatives of his choice free from restraint, interference, coercion, discrimination, or reprisal";

6. To manage his own personal finances, or to "be given at least a quarterly accounting of financial transactions made on his behalf should the facility accept his written delegation of this responsibility to the facility for any period of time in conformance with State law";

7. To be consistently "free from mental and physical abuse, and free from chemical and (except in emergencies) physical restraints except as authorized in writing by a physician for a specified and limited period of time or when necessary to protect the patient from injury to himself or others";

8. To be guaranteed confidentiality of all treatment and both medical and personal records and the assurance that these will not be released without his approval "except as required by law or third-party contract";

9. To be "treated with consideration, respect, and full recognition of his dignity and individuality, including privacy in treatment and in care for his personal needs";

10. To be assured that he will never be "required to perform services for the facility that are not included for therapeutic purpose in his plan of care";

11. To "associate and communicate privately with persons of his choice, and send and receive his personal mail unopened, unless medically contraindicated (as documented by his physician in his medical record)";

12. To meet with persons and groups of his choice and to participate in any commercial, religious, and community activities "unless medically contraindicated (as documented by his physician in his medical record)";

13. To keep and use all of his personal clothing and belongings "as space permits, unless to do so would infringe upon rights of other patients, and unless medically contraindicated (as documented by his physician in his medical record)"; and

14. "If married [to be] assured privacy for visits by his/her spouse; if both are in-patients in the facility, they are permitted to share a room, unless medically contraindicated (as documented by the attending physician in the medical record)."

Although I endorse all the items listed above, I'm going to amplify and/or comment on some of the points already listed and then suggest additional rights that the bill disregards.

Amplifications

I suggest the following in order of their listing:

3. I would add, the patient should have the right to be kept informed of his medical condition *in terms he can reasonably be expected to understand,* and the further right to expect reasonable continuity of care and to be informed by his physician or a delegate of his physician of

his continuing health care requirements following discharge.

4. I would add, the patient should have the right to know of any relationship of his facility to a hospital or other health-care institution insofar as his care is concerned. He should have the right to understand the reasons for his transferral to another facility when this is indicated. The institution to which the patient is to be transferred must first have accepted the patient for transfer. In the event of emergency transfer to a hospital (or in the case of death) the nearest relative or friend should be notified immediately, either by telephone or telegram.

5. The patient's right to voice grievances and recommend changes in policies and services is meaningless unless he understands lines of authority. For this purpose a copy of the nursing home's organizational chart should be posted in a public area easily accessible to all patients and available on request by patients who are bedridden.

Further, and apparently overlooked in the phrasing, if not the intent, of right No. 6 is the obvious fact that a patient's right to "voice grievances and recommend changes" is totally without impact unless he is guaranteed that his voice will be heard, that his grievances and recommendations will be listened to and duly considered by the appropriate department head(s) and/or administrator, and that he will be given a reasonable explanation for any negative response.

The recommendation that the patient speak freely without fear of reprisal, discrimination, etc., is infinitely more easily said than accomplished. If a patient makes a direct suggestion to a charge nurse that she institute an innovation in procedure or eliminate a policy that has become a habit over the course of years, fur is apt to fly. Not always, but sometimes. And it can be impossible to pinpoint small acts of discrimination, reprisal, and even negligence. Some-one has to be the first to be awakened in the morning, or the last to be given his supper tray, a routine dental ap-pointment must be canceled to accommodate an emer-gency, or the call-bell just couldn't be answered promptly because three were ringing at the same time. "Restraint, interference, coercion, discrimination or reprisal" need not be blatant and extreme; they can all be practiced quietly and unobtrusively.

In order to support the intent of right No. 6, to guaran-tee the patient freedom to voice his opinions *without fear*, and the assurance that he will be recognized and heard, I reemphasize the value and the potential of the patients' council (pages 44, 45). I would like to see the federal govern-ment mandate such a council in every long-term care facil-ity, establish guidelines for its composition and modus operandi and the requirement that it meet on a monthly basis. Responsibility should be placed on the administra-tor to submit regular written reports to the licensing agency covering (1) the minutes of each council meeting as submitted to him, (2) action taken as a result of each meeting, and (3) supportive reasons, and the explanation presented to patients for any administrative decisions to modify or to deny patient recommendations.

Were this to be a legal requirement for all long-term care facilities, the collective information gathered from pa-tients would present a new and meaningful basis for fu-ture planning of nursing homes: construction, program-ming, staffing, in-service education, patient-care policies, and almost every aspect of nursing-home care. All of us who work in the nursing-home field are accustomed to seminars, institutes, conferences, and what-have-you con-ducted among isolated groups of professionals: doctors, nurses, administrators, therapists, dietitians, architects, etc. These are held on county level, statewide, nationally, and internationally. The one group that has never been tapped as a trenchant source for identifying patients' needs, and reaching to meet them, is the most salient group—the patients themselves. Aggregate reports from monthly patients' council meetings throughout the nation would in large part eliminate professional guesswork, present an accurate and detailed picture of patient needs, and provide a reliable foundation for future long-term care.

6. I would add, the patient should have the right to expect that regular and frequent hours shall be established for cashing checks and for the disbursement of such monies or belongings of his as he may require on request. He should have the further right to receive and examine an explanation of his bill regardless of source of payment.

10. Although it may appear to you to be a farfetched provision that no patient be "required to perform services for the facility that are not included for therapeutic purpose in his plan of care," unfortunately, it is not. It is realistic in the extreme; and for that very reason I'd like to add "his plan of care as *as approved by his physician.*"

Within the confines of my personal experience I have not observed a nursing-home patient required to perform such services. However, I have been unhappily aware of such requirements practiced almost routinely in a number of mental hospitals. A friend of mine tells of a time when she was confined to a county mental hospital because of severe psychological depression. In that setting, during a time of dependence and suffering for all those who were institutionalized, if patients worked, they were rewarded. It was as simple as that. But the work was hard, and the rewards were diminutive. She tells of women who worked all day cleaning the homes of hospital executives who lived on the grounds. The women were paid 25 cents for the day's work. She herself worked from 8 A.M. until 5 P.M. as a waitress in the hospital's coffee shop. Her rewards were twofold: a pack of cigarettes each day and two meals in the coffee shop instead of standing on line in the patients' cafeteria.

The type of work and the long hours assigned prohibit the possibility of considering this practice within the realm of psychiatric or occupational therapy or instruction in the activities of daily living. A realistic approach provides the single answer that it was "free help."

Surely this sort of routine could extend into nursing homes and probably does. Thus I feel that right No. 10 is an important aspect to the patients' bill of rights.

11. Any "medical contraindication" to this right should be legally and specifically restricted to rare and extraordinary instances.

13. I would add, the patient should have the right to reasonable storage area for personal belongings and to a safe for the placement of his valuables; as well as the right to expect the institution to provide for the laundering and dry-cleaning of his personal clothing.

Additional Patients' Rights

It would be an almost superhuman task to enumerate all the rights of patients since these parallel the rights inherent to all human beings. Nevertheless, some of these patients' rights seem to me so compelling that I'm going to list them here as additions to the fourteen items set forth by the Department of Health, Education and Welfare.

The nursing home patient should have the further right:

15. To every consideration of his social needs. This shall include a full-time professionally directed recreation program with provision for outside trips unless medically con-

traindicated; a readily accessible outdoor area; an assortment of books, magazines, and games in good condition convenient for his use; religious services scheduled at least weekly, and a clergyman of the patient's faith on call for emergencies; and a planned program for introducing the patient to fellow patients and to staff members as soon as is medically feasible after admission. The patient has the further right to expect separate and equally salient programs for alert, senile, and bedridden patients, and the confidence that staff members are fully aware and equally respectful of the differing needs;

16. To use the facility as his home to as great an extent as possible. The patient has the right to elect his own bedtime unless medically prescribed; to have a comfortable chair and reading lamp in his bedroom; to go to a dining room for meals unless he is medically restricted; to be given good grooming care on a daily basis; to have escort service available to him when needed; and to have adequate instruction in the activities of daily living (ADL) whenever and as often as this is indicated. He has the right to expect that every effort shall be made to place him with suitable roommate(s); that visiting hours shall be liberal, and exceptions to those hours shall be made whenever possible for due cause; and that a sufficient number of public telephones shall be available for his use;

17. To such rehabilitative, consultative, and adjunct medical and dental services as his care may require; the right to know and understand the reason for each and the course of his progress, and the right to know in advance of appointment times;

18. To expect that at least one staff member shall be assigned primarily or solely to deal with the personal needs of the patients. This can be, but need not necessarily be, a trained social service worker;

19. To be insured optimal care through a well-planned and well-instructed continuing in-service education program for all members of the staff, regularly updated patient-care plans, regular meetings of the Patient Care Policies Committee, and routine interdepartmental meetings;

20. To a nurses' call-bell system that can be turned off only at his bedside;

21. To choice on his menu. This holds true even if his diet is medically restricted, in which case he has the further right to an understandable explanation of the restrictions;

22. To ample clean linens with as many changes as his particular condition may require for comfort and health;

23. To expect cleanliness, safety, and dependable maintenance of building, furnishings, and equipment.

24. To look forward to tomorrow.

Now that I conclude this chapter, it occurs to me that the patients' rights might have better constituted the preface, not just to this handbook, but to all the rules and regulations, the programs and personnel, and the purpose and concept of nursing homes everywhere.

Index